RESEARCH TRAINING IN PSYCHIATRY RESIDENCY

Strategies for Reform

Committee on Incorporating Research into Psychiatry Residency Training
Board on Neuroscience and Behavioral Health

Michael T. Abrams, Kathleen M. Patchan,
and Thomas F. Boat, *Editors*

INSTITUTE OF MEDICINE
OF THE NATIONAL ACADEMIES

THE NATIONAL ACADEMIES PRESS
Washington, D.C.
www.nap.edu

THE NATIONAL ACADEMIES PRESS   500 Fifth STREET, N.W.   Washington, DC 20001

NOTICE: The project that is the subject of this report was approved by the Governing Board of the National Research Council, whose members are drawn from the councils of the National Academy of Sciences, the National Academy of Engineering, and the Institute of Medicine. The members of the committee responsible for the report were chosen for their special competences and with regard for appropriate balance.

Support for this project was provided by the Institute of Mental Health. The views presented in this report are those of the Institute of Medicine Committee on Incorporating Research into Psychiatry Residency Training and are not necessarily those of the funding agencies.

International Standard Book Number 0-309-09071-7
International Standard Book Number 0-309-52741-4 (PDF)

Additional copies of this report are available from the National Academies Press, 500 Fifth Street, N.W., Lockbox 285, Washington, DC 20055; (800) 624-6242 or (202) 334-3313 (in the Washington metropolitan area); Internet, http://www.nap.edu.

For more information about the Institute of Medicine, visit the IOM home page at: **www.iom.edu.**

Copyright 2003 by the National Academy of Sciences. All rights reserved.

Printed in the United States of America.

The serpent has been a symbol of long life, healing, and knowledge among almost all cultures and religions since the beginning of recorded history. The serpent adopted as a logotype by the Institute of Medicine is a relief carving from ancient Greece, now held by the Staatliche Museen in Berlin.

Cover art: "The Thinker" by Brian S. McQuillan

*"Knowing is not enough; we must apply.
Willing is not enough; we must do."*
—Goethe

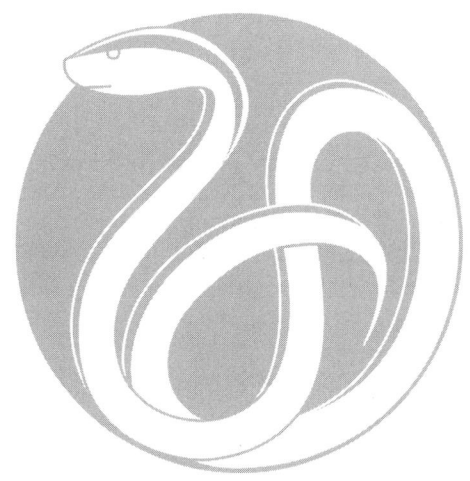

INSTITUTE OF MEDICINE
OF THE NATIONAL ACADEMIES

Shaping the Future for Health

THE NATIONAL ACADEMIES
Advisers to the Nation on Science, Engineering, and Medicine

The **National Academy of Sciences** is a private, nonprofit, self-perpetuating society of distinguished scholars engaged in scientific and engineering research, dedicated to the furtherance of science and technology and to their use for the general welfare. Upon the authority of the charter granted to it by the Congress in 1863, the Academy has a mandate that requires it to advise the federal government on scientific and technical matters. Dr. Bruce M. Alberts is president of the National Academy of Sciences.

The **National Academy of Engineering** was established in 1964, under the charter of the National Academy of Sciences, as a parallel organization of outstanding engineers. It is autonomous in its administration and in the selection of its members, sharing with the National Academy of Sciences the responsibility for advising the federal government. The National Academy of Engineering also sponsors engineering programs aimed at meeting national needs, encourages education and research, and recognizes the superior achievements of engineers. Dr. Wm. A. Wulf is president of the National Academy of Engineering.

The **Institute of Medicine** was established in 1970 by the National Academy of Sciences to secure the services of eminent members of appropriate professions in the examination of policy matters pertaining to the health of the public. The Institute acts under the responsibility given to the National Academy of Sciences by its congressional charter to be an adviser to the federal government and, upon its own initiative, to identify issues of medical care, research, and education. Dr. Harvey V. Fineberg is president of the Institute of Medicine.

The **National Research Council** was organized by the National Academy of Sciences in 1916 to associate the broad community of science and technology with the Academy's purposes of furthering knowledge and advising the federal government. Functioning in accordance with general policies determined by the Academy, the Council has become the principal operating agency of both the National Academy of Sciences and the National Academy of Engineering in providing services to the government, the public, and the scientific and engineering communities. The Council is administered jointly by both Academies and the Institute of Medicine. Dr. Bruce M. Alberts and Dr. Wm. A. Wulf are chair and vice chair, respectively, of the National Research Council.

www.national-academies.org

COMMITTEE ON INCORPORATING RESEARCH INTO PSYCHIATRY RESIDENCY TRAINING

THOMAS F. BOAT (*Chair*), Chairman, Department of Pediatrics, University of Cincinnati, Ohio
BARBARA F. ATKINSON, Dean, School of Medicine, University of Kansas, Kansas City
BENJAMIN S. BUNNEY, Charles BG Murphy Professor and Chairman, Department of Psychiatry, Yale University, New Haven, Connecticut
GABRIELLE A. CARLSON, Director, Child Psychiatry, State University of New York at Stony Brook, New York
JAMES J. HUDZIAK, Director, Child Psychiatry, University of Vermont, Burlington
DEAN G. KILPATRICK, Professor, Psychiatry and Behavioral Sciences, Medical University of South Carolina, Charleston
WILLIAM B. LAWSON, Professor and Chair of Psychiatry, Howard University, Washington, D.C.
VIRGINIA MAN-YEE LEE, Co-Director, Center of Neurodegenerative Disease Research, University of Pennsylvania, Philadelphia
JEROME B. POSNER, George Cotzias Chair, Neuro-Oncology, Memorial Sloan-Kettering Cancer Center, New York
MICHELLE B. RIBA, Associate Chair, Department of Psychiatry, University of Michigan Medical Center, Ann Arbor
RICHARD M. SCHEFFLER, Professor, School of Public Health, University of California, Berkeley
JOEL YAGER, Professor and Vice Chair for Education, University of New Mexico, Albuquerque

Board on Neuroscience and Behavioral Health Liaison

DAVID REISS, Professor, Psychiatry, George Washington University, Washington, D.C.

Study Staff

MICHAEL T. ABRAMS, Study Director
KATHLEEN M. PATCHAN, Research Assistant (from October 2002)
MILAP NOWRANGI, Research Assistant (January-July 2002)
BRIAN S. McQUILLAN, Senior Project Assistant (December 2001-October 2002)
PARISA MORRIS, Christine Mirzayan Intern (June-August 2002)

Board on Neuroscience and Behavioral Health Staff

ANDREW M. POPE, Acting Director
TERRY C. PELLMAR, Director (until October 2002)
JANET JOY, Senior Program Officer
MICHAEL T. ABRAMS, Program Officer
LAUREN HONESS-MORREALE, Program Officer
LYNN NIELSEN-BOHLMAN, Program Officer
PATRICIA CUFF, Research Associate
ALLISON M. PANZER, Research Assistant
KATHLEEN M. PATCHAN, Research Assistant
LORA K. TAYLOR, Senior Project Assistant
ALLISON BERGER, Project Assistant
ROSA POMMIER, Finance Officer

INDEPENDENT REPORT REVIEWERS

This report has been reviewed in draft form by individuals chosen for their diverse perspectives and technical expertise, in accordance with procedures approved by the NRC's Report Review Committee. The purpose of this independent review is to provide candid and critical comments that will assist the institution in making its published report as sound as possible and to ensure that the report meets institutional standards for objectivity, evidence, and responsiveness to the study charge. The review comments and draft manuscript remain confidential to protect the integrity of the deliberative process. We wish to thank the following individuals for their review of this report:

Joseph D. Bloom, Oregon Health Services University, School of Medicine
Veronica M. Catanese, New York University School of Medicine
Mina K. Dulcan, Northwestern University, Feinberg School of Medicine
Larry D. Gruppen, University of Michigan Medical School
Lewis L. Judd, University of California, San Diego School of Medicine
Jeffrey A. Lieberman, University of North Carolina School of Medicine
Georgine M. Pion, Vanderbilt Institute for Public Policy Studies
Ronald O. Rieder, Columbia University, and New York State Psychiatric Institute
Stephen C. Scheiber, American Board of Psychiatry and Neurology
Charles B. Wilson, Health Technology Center, and the University of California, San Francisco

Although the reviewers listed above have provided many constructive comments and suggestions, they were not asked to endorse the conclusions or recommendations nor did they see the final draft of the report before its release. The review of this report was overseen by **David N. Sundwall**, American Clinical Laboratory Association, and **Henry W. Riecken**, University of Pennsylvania. Appointed by the National Research Council and the Institute of Medicine, they were responsible for making certain that an independent examination of this report was carried out in accordance with institutional procedures and that all review comments were carefully considered. Responsibility for the final content of this report rests entirely with the authoring committee and the institution.

Preface

Large numbers of individuals are in need of treatment and support for mental disorders. At the same time, the capacity of the health care system to support caregivers and other resources has lagged behind the demand for services. Over the decades, outcomes for individuals with serious behavioral problems have improved, but much needs to be done to meet current needs.

Strategic initiatives to meet this challenge include improving care systems, as well as improving modalities of care—diagnostic, therapeutic, and preventive. Ultimately, new modalities of care will be required to ensure a more effective and efficient mental health care system. Opportunities for improvement through research have never been greater. Research tools, both biological and clinical, are increasingly applicable to a wide range of mental health questions and problems. Rapid advances in understanding the biological and functional basis for behavior and its alterations promise to spawn creative and effective clinical insights.

The National Institute of Mental Health sponsored this study of research training in psychiatry residency because of a growing concern that the numbers of psychiatrist-investigators have been falling short of meeting the need and the opportunities to advance the field. This concern is particularly acute in the area of child and adolescent psychiatry. NIMH, while certainly eager to stimulate relevant efforts in biological discovery, was particularly eager to focus this study on efforts directed at training of patient-oriented investigators.

The study committee, convened by the Institute of Medicine at the request of NIMH, gathered relevant information from many sources, but soon recognized that evidence available for assessing the magnitude of perceived problems in psychiatric research training and for devising potential solutions is limited. In addition, the committee's assessment was complicated by several factors: (1) much psychiatric research is carried out by Ph.D. scientists as well as by psychiatrist-investigators; (2) psychiatry is less uniformly oriented to standard treatment approaches than are other specialties; and (3) the charge to the committee was to focus on research in core residency training, a segment of training that has traditionally had the objective of ensuring clinical rather than research competency.

Recognizing the challenge inherent in its assignment, the committee resolutely considered a broad range of salient information in formulating a set of recommendations that reflect current evidence, as well as numerous carefully considered opinions. Among its recommendations, the committee in particular calls for a more cohesive approach by the psychiatry community to the issue of research training of psychiatrists, which as a first step would include assembly of a broadly representative national body to implement and further craft strategies to ensure more successful recruitment and training of psychiatrists for productive research careers. Thus, the committee hopes its efforts will be taken up by a steering group empowered to monitor and make future improvements to the training of psychiatrist-investigators as needed to advance psychiatric practice.

I would like to thank all the members of the committee for spirited discussions tempered by a sense of purpose, including a uniformly perceived need to present a call for action. I am certain that all the members join me in expressing deep appreciation to Michael Abrams, whose insights, determination, and persistence were key factors in translating a large volume of information and opinions into a cohesive report.

Finally, I wish to acknowledge the contribution of a few individuals who offered "behind the scenes" assistance to the completion of this report. Manuscript review and senior-level project support were furnished by Gooloo Wunderlich, Andy Pope, Melvin Worth, Douglas Weil, and Terry Pellmar. Detailed editing of the full report was provided by Rona Briere, while Margie Patlak provided some useful science writing. Finally, Sharon Turner and Judy Estep both offered important meeting planning and production support in the late stages of the study. Other contributors to this study are acknowledged throughout the text or listed in appendix A. In short, this report could not have been completed without the generous cooperation of a great number of competent individuals.

Thomas F. Boat
Chair

Contents

Executive Summary   1

1   Introduction   21
Study Context, 21
    The Burden of Mental Illness, 21
    Increasing Societal Awareness of Mental Illness, 22
    Advances in Mental Health Care, 22
Genesis of the Study, 25
    Trends in Training of Psychiatrist-Researchers, 25
    Study Charge, 29
    Composition of the Committee, 30
Study Approach and Scope, 30
    Overall Strategy, 30
    Definitions and Broad Concepts, 30
    Limitations of the Data, 34
Organization of the Report, 34

2   Residency as Part of a Longitudinal Career Continuum   37
Residency as an Important Target for Research Training, 37
    Research Literacy, 39
    Exposures and Experiences, 40
    Opportunities to Formulate Patient-Oriented Research
        Questions, 42
    Attracting and Sustaining the Interest of Talented Medical
        Students, 42
Importance of Longitudinal Training for Potential Researchers, 43
    Preresidency Experiences, 44
    Postresidency Experiences, 47
Strategic Considerations, 54
    Models from Outside of Psychiatry, 55
Conclusions and Recommendation 2.1, 58

3 Regulatory Factors   61

Psychiatry Residency Review Committee, 61
    Organization and Function, 61
    A Brief Detour into Psychodynamic Psychotherapy, 64
    Clinical Requirements for Psychiatry Training, 68
    Other Opportunities for Research Experiences in Residency, 75
    Research Requirements for Psychiatric Residency, 77
Certification Board, American Board of Psychiatry and Neurology, 80
American Medical Association, 82
Other National Organizations Involved in Psychiatric Research Training, 82
    American Psychiatric Association, 82
    American Academy of Child and Adolescent Psychiatry, 83
    Other National Organizations, 84
Conclusions and Recommendations, 84

4 Institutional Factors   91

Funding Issues in Graduate Medical Education, 91
    The General Funding Stream, 91
    Funding Issues in Pediatric Graduate Medical Education, 93
    Supporting Research Activity Through Graduate Medical Education Funds, 93
    General Research Funding, 95
Leadership and Mentoring, 102
    Institutional Leadership, 102
    Departmental Leadership, 104
    Mentorship, 105
Program and Curriculum Structure, 109
    Published Reports on Research Curriculum Design, 109
    Illustrative Programs, 114
    Other Aggregate Program Data, 120
Conclusions and Recommendations, 125

5 Personal Factors   133

Innate Characteristics, 133
    Motivation and Drive, 134
    Intellectual Capacity and Scientific Orientation, 134
Personal Financial Concerns, 138
    Student Debt, 138
    Residency and Fellowship Stipends, 139

Salaries of Psychiatrists Compared with Other Specialties, 139
Salary Differences Between Clinicians and Researchers, 141
Nonsalary Benefits of a Research Career, 144
Representation of Women, International Medical Graduates, and Racial Minorities in Psychiatry, 150
Women, 152
International Medical Graduates, 154
Underrepresented Racial and Ethnic Minorities, 156
Conclusions and Recommendations, 159

6 Future Directions for Promoting the Development of Psychiatrist-Researchers   167
Workforce Estimates and Monitoring, 167
Outcome Data in Research Training, 171
National Coordinating Effort, 173
Overarching Recommendation, 174

References   177

Appendix A: Data Sources and Methods   201

Appendix B: Federal and Other Funding Mechanisms Listed and Summarized by Career Stage   211

Appendix C: Brief Descriptions of Psychiatry Residency Training Programs   231

Appendix D: Committee and Staff Biographies   247

Tables, Figures, and Boxes

TABLES

ES-1 Summary of Recommendations, 19
1-1   Research Involvement Rates of Practicing Psychiatrists, 27
2-1   Western Psychiatric Institute and Clinic's Developmental Pathways for Psychiatric Researchers, 55
2-2   Duration in Years of the Two Stages of Pediatric Subspecialty Training Pathways, 57
3-1   Summary of Duration, Time, and Research Requirements for Accredited Residency Training Programs, 70–71
4-1   Sources of Graduate Medical Education Funding, 92
4-2   Research Training Outcome Data from Several Residency Programs in Psychiatry, 124
4-3   Continuum of Residency-Based Research Training, 131
5-1   Examination Scores by Specialty Choice upon Entry to Medical School (MCAT) and upon Entry to Residency (USMLE), 136
5-2   Median Expected Starting Income for Graduates of New York State and California Residency Training Programs, 2002, 140
5-3   Selected Data from the American Psychiatric Association's 1998 National Survey of Psychiatric Practice, 143
5-4   Demographic Composition of Residents in Various Specialties or Subspecialties of Medicine, 151

FIGURES

1-1   Percent of National Institute of Mental Health (NIMH) extramural grants stratified by the five major disciplines, 26
2-1   Training pathways in psychiatry, 38

5-1 Ratio of demand to supply of medical students who designate a given residency as their first career choice, versus the expected lifetime income, 141
5-2 Percent of National Institute of Mental Health (NIMH) research project grants that were awarded to principal investigators, stratified by highest degree, 148
5-3 Success rate of National Institute of Mental Health (NIMH) research project grant applications, stratified by degree of the principal investigator, 149
5-4 Total number (table) and percentage (graph) of all, female, and international medical graduate (IMGs) physicians declaring research as their primary activity, 1970–2000, 152
5-5 Number of international medical graduates (IMG) and U.S. medical graduates who entered psychiatry as PGY1 residents, 155

BOXES

2-1 Rationale for Incorporating Research Training into the Residency Experience, 38
3-1 Requirements Prescribed by the Psychiatry Residency Review Committee for Accredited Programs in Adult (General) Psychiatry, 73
3-2 Requirements Prescribed by the Psychiatry Residency Review Committee for Accredited Programs in Child and Adolescent Psychiatry, 74
3-3 Summary of Topics Included on Written Portion of Psychiatry Board Examination, 81
5-1 Nonsalary Benefits of a Research Career, 144
6-1 Three Studies Suggesting the Need for Psychiatrist-Researchers, 170–171

Executive Summary

Abstract: *The neural and behavioral sciences have advanced tremendously in recent years, and there has been a concomitant increase in public awareness of mental disorders. Psychiatrists are on the front line of treating mental illness. Some psychiatrists also serve as patient-oriented researchers, advancing psychiatric care through investigation aimed at helping those with or at risk for mental disorders. Unfortunately, the number of psychiatrist-researchers does not appear to be keeping pace with the unparalleled needs that currently exist in clinical brain and behavioral medicine. The need is especially acute in child and adolescent psychiatry. In this context, the National Institute of Mental Health asked the Institute of Medicine (IOM) to convene a committee to study research training during psychiatric residency. The IOM committee was charged with considering (1) the goals of psychiatric residency training, (2) programs that train researchers successfully, (3) obstacles to efficient research training, and (4) strategies for overcoming those obstacles.*

The committee found that significant influences on research training span three major conceptual categories: regulatory, institutional, and personal factors. Cutting across these factors are the ubiquitous and overlapping issues of time and money, and the competing demands of patient-care activities. A considerable time investment—2 to 4 years—beyond core clinical training is typically required for successful research training. Therefore, the committee concluded that more and better residency-based research training may have the important and dual benefits of optimizing the length of training for, and solidifying research career interests of, greater numbers of junior psychiatrists.

Regarding regulatory factors, a review of the psychiatry residency accreditation requirements led the committee to conclude that these requirements should be modified to afford more training time for research experiences and general research literacy. Institutional factors of greatest importance were found to be supportive leadership and the involve-

ment *of research faculty as residency educators and mentors. A review of personal factors revealed motivation and drive, family demands, gender, and race as important factors relevant to research training in psychiatry. This finding led the committee to conclude that a more diverse group of trainees needs to be persuaded that research careers in psychiatry are worthwhile. Greater financial incentives (through stipend supplements or debt repayment) and more aggressive promotion of the benefits of participation in psychiatric research are recommended as strategies to enhance trainee recruitment.*

In addition to time and money, overarching themes of this report are that residency-based research is limited because of the demands of clinical training, and thus that successful research training typically requires the linkage of residency to postresidency research fellowships. There is little evidence to support any particular approach to training patient-oriented investigators. Given that the existence of a large research effort (i.e., many investigators and substantial funding) is the most salient feature of successful programs, child and adolescent psychiatry divisions and small programs in general will likely require outside collaborations to develop a critical mass of resources for effective research training. Finally, while there are numerous efforts under way to enhance research training in psychiatric residency, the committee recommends the formation of a national coordinating body to develop, implement, and evaluate strategies toward that goal.

STUDY CONTEXT

Mental disorders, such as schizophrenia, severe depression or anxiety, and substance abuse, represent some of the most debilitating and vexing of human diseases. Recent years have seen considerable advances in the brain and behavioral sciences, but the burden of mental disorders remains very high, accounting for approximately 15 percent of all human disease (Murray and Lopez, 1996). Understanding of the mechanisms underlying such disorders is expanding at a tremendous rate, but remains limited compared with the vast complexity of human neurobiology and behavior (Charney et al., 2001; Kandel et al., 2000). Carefully formulated research in a variety of disciplines is clearly needed to accelerate progress in mental health care, and this research needs to be skillfully aimed at questions relevant to patients who suffer from or are at risk for mental disorders.

Research Involvement of Psychiatrists

By virtue of their medical school and clinical residency training, psychiatrists have expertise in the diagnosis and treatment of serious mental disorders and in the neurobiological basis of these disorders. It therefore appears obvious that they would be interested in and capable of contributing to the mental health research effort. Yet while many psychiatrists conduct research, a 1989 survey found that only 15 percent of psychiatrists *who are faculty at U.S. medical schools* spent more than half of their professional time engaged in research (Pincus et al., 1993), and more recent surveys conducted in 1999 and 2000 showed that fewer than 2 percent of *all* U.S. psychiatrists consider research their dominant activity (Association of American Medical Colleges [AAMC], 2002b). Data from the American Psychiatric Association (APA) indicate that, along with these low baseline rates of research involvement, research fellowships to train young psychiatrists appear to be on the decline (APA, 1997a; Fenton, 2002; Guerra and Regier, 2001; Nevin and Pincus, 1992; Steele and Pincus, 1995). Overall, then, research training and research involvement by psychiatrists appear to be limited and may be decreasing (Fenton, 2002; Halpain et al., 2001; Hyman, 2002b; Kupfer et al., 2002).

Genesis of the Study and the Study Charge

The National Institute of Mental Health (NIMH) is at the center of U.S. efforts to advance mental health and is a principal source of funding for psychiatrist trainees and established researchers. In 2001, NIMH awarded $230 million in education and research grants to psychiatrist-investigators (data furnished by NIMH, Office of Science Policy and Program Policy, February 21, 2003). NIMH believes the number of psychiatrist-researchers is not keeping pace with the increased funding and unparalleled opportunities that exist in patient-oriented mental health research (Fenton, 2002; Hyman and Fenton, 2003; Shore et al., 2001). As part of a larger strategy to address this problem, NIMH asked the Institute of Medicine (IOM) to convene an expert committee that would evaluate the current goals of psychiatry residency training and consider strategies for enhancing research training during or in close proximity to residency. Specifically, the IOM committee was asked to address the following four issues in the context of adult, and child and adolescent psychiatric residency: (1) the goals of training, with an emphasis on both core research training and training trajectories to facilitate patient-oriented research career development; (2) programs that successfully train patient-oriented researchers; (3) obstacles to efficient research training at both research-intensive and other institutions, and (4) strategies for overcoming those obstacles.

CONCLUSIONS AND RECOMMENDATIONS

Before presenting the recommendations of this report the committee must caution readers that data regarding both the magnitude of the problem, and the effectiveness of proposed solutions, were limited. Limitations stemmed from a number of sources. First, it is challenging to estimate the physician workforce across medical specialties (Council on Graduate Medical Education [COGME], 2000). Second, in psychiatry and most medical disciplines there are many non-physician investigators who make invaluable contributions to clinical research, therefore, workforce estimates are further complicated by considering those experts (Fang and Meyer, 2003). Finally, documentation of residency-based clinical research education is scarce and often imprecise thereby inhibiting extensive and objective evaluation (Hebert et al., 2003; Sheets and Anderson, 1991). Because of these limitations, the committee drew heavily from its collective expertise and experience in making its recommendations.

Through a review of the existing literature, as well as numerous personal contacts, the committee identified the need to place residency in the broad longitudinal continuum of physician training—from the undergraduate years, to medical school, residency, fellowship, and beyond—when addressing research training needs for psychiatry residents. The committee also identified three distinct sets of factors that influence research training during or in close proximity to psychiatric residency:

• *Regulatory factors*, comprising program accreditation and individual certification requirements that are governed by the Psychiatry Residency Review Committee (RRC) under the auspices of the Accreditation Council for Graduate Medical Education (ACGME) and by the American Board of Psychiatry and Neurology (ABPN). Both the Psychiatry RRC and the ABPN are independent, not-for-profit bodies that have historically placed much greater emphasis on clinical than on research training issues.

• *Institutional factors*, encompassing the research and research-training milieu of individual residency programs. The training environment comprises curriculum, departmental and institutional faculty and

leadership, facilities and finances, and the existing portfolio of ongoing research projects.
- *Personal factors*, including innate ability and drive, educational debt, family responsibilities, race, and gender.

Finally, the cross-cutting issues of time, money, and clinical demands relate to and even transcend many of the above factors. Clinical demands are especially pertinent because residents need to diagnose and treat patients as a means of gaining practical experience, and because patient needs are often more urgent than patient-oriented research.

Residency as Part of a Continuum of Training

Central to program infrastructure are the duration and timing of research training. After careful consideration of research training in the context of residency, the committee concluded that psychiatry residency is a pivotal interval during which preliminary research training should be offered. It represents an opportunity to (1) prepare all residents for the lifelong practice of evidence-based medicine (Mulrow and Lohr, 2001; Sackett et al., 1996), (2) provide some residents with initial research experiences that may launch them into a patient-oriented research career, and (3) sustain the research interests of trainees with previous research experience (e.g., M.D./Ph.D.'s). That having been said, the committee also concluded that postresidency fellowship training is required to give medical trainees the skills and knowledge needed to embark on a career as an independent, productive researcher.

Fellowship training beyond residency is important preparation for a sustained career in research, both within and outside of psychiatry (Davis and Kelley, 1982; Dial et al., 1990; Dunn et al., 1998; Haviland et al., 1987; Pincus et al., 1993; Ringel et al., 2001). These fellowships take place immediately after residency and last 1 to 3 years. Internal medicine, pediatrics, and other medical specialties rely on extended research training and typically couple it with subspecialty training. By contrast, psychiatry seems to have developed subspecialty tracks (e.g., geriatrics) which do not usually include substantive research training goals. The more research-intensive departments in psychiatry place heavy emphasis on offering research fellowships and on connecting those fellowships to core residency training, but most training programs in psychiatry do not appear to facilitate such connectivity. To foster this connectivity between residency and research fellowships in psychiatry, the committee makes the following recommendation:

Recommendation 2.1.[1] **Departments of psychiatry should organize optional research experiences and mandatory research didactics in residency as early steps in research career development pathways, leading from residency to a junior faculty appointment. Federal and private agencies should expand mechanisms that encourage psychiatry trainees to enter and move, without interruption, from residency to a research fellowship to a faculty position, all designed to promote independence as a patient-oriented investigator.**

Regulatory Factors

The two regulatory bodies with the greatest influence over psychiatry residency training are the ABPN and the Psychiatry RRC. These two bodies aim to safeguard consumer health by ensuring that all residency graduates are competent to deliver quality psychiatric care. The ABPN certifies individuals, through an examination process that occurs after residency has been completed, while the RRC mandates minimal standards to which programs must adhere to be accredited to train future psychiatrists. A review of the RRC requirements for adult and for child and adolescent psychiatry led the committee to conclude that the clinical requirements could be reduced to foster greater flexibility in training that might include offering research training electives (ACGME, 2000a; 2000b). This reduction would involve limiting some of the timed and untimed requirements that have been added in recent years. For example, the psychotherapy requirement, which includes the achievement of competency in five broad areas, could be reduced to knowledge in those five areas and competency in a subset. Additionally, inpatient service of 9 months could be reduced to 6 months to allow time for other experiences. Given the apparent universal belief that protected time for research activity is critical for research success (Costa et al., 2000; DeHaven et al., 1998; Griggs, 2002; McGuire and Fairbanks, 1982; Raphael et al., 1990; Roberts and Bogenschutz, 2001; Schrier, 1997; Shine, 1998; Shore et al., 2001), the committee makes the following recommendation:

---

[1] For ease of reference, the committee's recommendations are numbered according to the chapter of the main text in which they appear followed by the order in which they appear in that chapter.

Recommendation 3.1. The American Board of Psychiatry and Neurology and the Psychiatry Residency Review Committee should make the requirements for board certification and residency accreditation more flexible so research training can occur during residency at a level that significantly increases the probability of more residents choosing research as a career. The committee further recommends that residents who successfully fulfill core requirements at an accelerated pace, with competency being used as the measure, be allowed to spend the time thus made available to pursue research training.

The ABPN and the Psychiatry RRC should provide written guidelines and ongoing support to assist programs in incorporating research experiences into all years of residency. This recommendation is aimed at optimizing core training by streamlining some of the redundant or overly ambitious requirements of that training, and by permitting programs and individuals the opportunity to tailor larger portions of their training with elective experiences that might include "hands-on" research activity. The recommendation further aims to entice outstanding residents to undertake research activity by rewarding fast-paced attainment of clinical competency with greater opportunities for early research involvement. Implementation of this recommendation will depend on enabling guidelines from both the RRC and the ABPN. This recommendation is consistent with an ACGME initiative aimed at competency-based rather than time-based training (ACGME, 2002b).

While the committee advocates increased flexibility in clinical requirements, we also conclude that the research requirements of residency training should be strengthened to facilitate the field's progression as an evidence-based discipline (Mulrow and Lohr, 2001; Sackett et al., 1996). Although the requirements of the Psychiatry RRC do characterize research experiences and didactics as clear "shoulds," most programs appear to offer very little in the way of research training for their residents (Balon and Singh, 2001). Even the strongest programs usually delay research exposure until the last 2 years of the residency. Accordingly, the committee makes the following recommendation:

Recommendation 3.2. The American Board of Psychiatry and Neurology and the Psychiatry Residency Review Committee should require patient-oriented

> research literacy as a core competency of residency training in adult and child and adolescent psychiatry. Program directors and the American Board of Psychiatry and Neurology should evaluate residents on these competencies.

This recommendation should be implemented by strengthening the language of the current Psychiatry RRC requirements to indicate that all curricula must address research design and methods as preparation for the lifelong practice of evidence-based medicine. The ABPN should enforce the requirement for literacy in patient-oriented research by adding more questions on research to the certification examination. Content for program didactics and for the examination in the context of residency training could come from any number of published works on clinical research in general or in psychiatry in particular (Blazer and Hays, 1998). A review of various published curricula indicates that research literacy in psychiatry should include knowledge in at least the following areas: epidemiology, study design, biostatistics, integrated clinical neural and behavioral science, research ethics, and grant and manuscript writing skills. This knowledge could be addressed by adding content to the in-training and credentialing examinations that are a standard part of psychiatrists' transition to independent practice.

Since expertise will be needed to craft guidelines for the competencies noted above, the following recommendation is important:

> **Recommendation 3.3. The organizations that nominate members for the Psychiatry Residency Review Committee and the American Board of Psychiatry and Neurology should include on their nomination lists substantial numbers of extramurally funded, experienced psychiatrist-investigators who conduct patient-oriented research.**

Research experience is not currently an explicit requirement for nomination to serve on the RRC or the ABPN. It is the committee's view that at least some of the slots on those regulatory bodies should be filled with skilled patient-oriented researchers. Doing so would greatly increase the probability that accreditation and certification policies will reflect the input of knowledgeable patient-oriented researchers. Implementation of this recommendation could be effected by one or more of the nominating bodies (e.g., American Psychiatric Association, American Medical Association) or by a change in the nomination policies of the ACGME (the umbrella organization for all RRCs) and the ABPN to mandate the inclusion of a certain number of patient-oriented researchers (ACGME, 2002c). As researchers are a small minority of all psychiatrists, a key constraint on the implementation of this recommendation is the willingness of researchers to commit some time to the educational mission. To facilitate that willingness, leaders in psychiatry should consider how to make such service responsibilities tenable. For example, service on the ABPN executive board requires a commitment of 45 days per year (personal communication, S. Scheiber, ABPN, April 5, 2003). Such a service requirement could be impossible for someone responsible for an ongoing research program unless his/her department chair (or extramural funding agency) offered some reprieve or extension on existing obligations, or unless the ABPN could devise some way to reduce the time commitment of key contributors.

Finally, it should be emphasized that, while RRC and ABPN policies clearly set standards for the entire field, these organizations are not directly responsible for clinical or research training. Local institutions are in charge of such training. If they are going to be successful at training new researchers, the individual programs themselves must strive to provide the necessary resources and opportunities, including research time, mentors, and a culture that genuinely supports and values the importance of generating new clinical knowledge.

Institutional Factors

Training Resources

Issues associated with funding, mentoring, and resident scheduling appear to be the chief constraints on research training in residency. Support for residency training is heavily dependent on Medicare funding for graduate medical education. That funding stream is under increasing pressure as federal and private payers seek ways to minimize health care costs. Research is not generally considered part of core residency training. As a result, funding for research activity often needs to be independently justified and obtained either from extramural grants or from discretionary internal funds (e.g., endowments, profits from practice plans). Furthermore, leadership at medical centers have control over how funds are distributed and they set expectations regarding trainee and faculty activity through institutional mechanisms such as promotion policies and general resource allocation. Therefore, the committee believes the following recommendation is critical to research training in psychiatry:

> **Recommendation 4.1. The broad psychiatry community should work more aggressively to encourage university presidents, deans and hospital chief executive officers to give greater priority to the advancement of mental health through investments in leadership, faculty, and infrastructure for research and research training in psychiatry departments.**

Although this recommendation is likely relevant to other branches of medical research, psychiatric research is of particular importance in this regard. This is the case because current opportunities in brain and behavioral research are so great, and because mental illness is the object of stigma and cost containment efforts that impede access to care as well as equitable reimbursement for mental health services (U. S. Department of Health and Human Services [DHHS], 1999; Frank et al., 2001b). Department chairs and other leaders could promote psychiatric research by developing a business case delineating the financial and societal benefits likely to result from mental health research. At the same time, these leaders should also inform medical students and residents regarding the extraordinary intellectual challenges that accompany research in psychiatry.

Mentoring is the ingredient cited most frequently as necessary for effective research training (Balon and Singh, 2001; DeHaven et al., 1998; IOM, 1994; Pincus et al., 1995). Limits on mentoring are also frequently noted as a barrier to effective research training (Lewinsohn et al., 1998). A logical extension of this observation is that more incentives are needed to encourage senior researchers to act as mentors to the next generation of research psychiatrists. Accordingly, the committee makes the following recommendation:

> **Recommendation 4.2. Academic institutions and their psychiatry residency training programs should reward the involvement of patient-oriented research faculty in the residency training process. The National Institute of Mental Health should take the lead in identifying funding mechanisms to support such incentives.**

This recommendation targets in particular smaller institutions with limited research programs that are likely to have difficulty attracting the most research-minded applicants seeking the most varied research training experience available. Such programs will be less competitive in attracting trainees with prior research experience, so that greater training and supervision will be required before their residents can extend the productivity of research mentors. Especially for less research-intensive programs, the committee encourages mechanisms to cover the additional mentoring costs associated with training research-naive residents. When on-site mentoring is not possible, a remote network (e.g., via the Internet) might be developed to give trainees the opportunity to reach beyond their home institution for scientific and career advice. At a minimum, such a network might assist residents with transient issues by providing occasional consultations; in some instances, however, it could lead residents to research fellowships or other even longer-term research collaborations with senior investigators. Senior researchers might be willing to act as remote mentors for a consulting fee and/or for the opportunity to establish collaborative or trainee recruitment links outside their institutions.

Development of Research Curricula

In addition to institutional leadership and mentoring, the committee reviewed generic clinical research training programs and several set specifically in the context of the psychiatric residency. These programs are highly variable. Generic programs range from 1-year certificates to multiyear programs that culminate with a Ph.D. degree. Although this range appears to be geared in part toward the broad mix of applicants, an AAMC task force concluded that such program variability in general reflects imprecision regarding the formal constitution of clinical research training (AAMC, 1999).

Common practices are nevertheless apparent from a review of existing programs and published descriptions. Most programs offer some research training in the later years of residency, and the most research-intensive institutions route their research-oriented graduates toward additional training, usually in the form of a fellowship. Hands-on research participation is encouraged. Course subject matter typically includes epidemiology, grant and paper writing, integrated neural and behavioral science, and research ethics. Little has been done to integrate substantial research training into all or even most of the residency years (Balon and Singh, 2001). Additionally, existing curricula typically are not validated by long-term follow-up studies to determine whether trainees were actually prepared to move into patient-oriented research careers or even to practice evidence-based medicine more efficiently. Given that it was difficult for the committee to identify truly successful programs beyond reputation, we make the following recommendation:

> **Recommendation 4.3. The National Institute of Mental Health, foundations, and other funding agencies should provide resources to support efforts to create competency-based curricula for research literacy and more comprehensive research training in psychiatry that are applicable across the spectrum of adult (general) and child and adolescent residency training programs. Supported curriculum development efforts should include plans for educating faculty to deliver each new curriculum, as well as plans for evaluating each curriculum's success in training individuals to competency and in recruiting and training successful researchers.**

These curricula should be aimed at sparking residents' interest in a lifelong career in patient-oriented research without interfering with core clinical training. The principal aim of this recommendation, however, is to ensure that all residents are adequately introduced to the concepts of research and that research training is not merely an afterthought to residency education. Thus the recommendation is focused on ensuring that all residency programs offer training that can contribute to the expansion of a patient-oriented research effort in psychiatry. Even residents who intend to become clinicians should be introduced to the concepts and findings of patient-oriented research as a necessary complement to their clinical training. Curricula should be developed using established educational principles; it is especially important to include evaluation phases to verify the utility of the curricula in the training of patient-oriented psychiatrist-researchers and evidence-based practitioners (Sheets and Anderson, 1991). Novel ways to integrate research training into the residency experience should also be considered.

The committee believes that, since psychiatric training programs vary considerably in terms of size and local expertise, they should be viewed along a hierarchical research training continuum that ranges from those providing basic research literacy to those training large numbers of patient-oriented psychiatrist-researchers. This continuum (detailed in the full report) can be used as a guide for programs interested in moving to a higher level of research training. It can also be used to implement the following recommendation, which is aimed at encouraging targeted

NIMH extramural support for the emergence of new mid- and high-range centers of excellence in patient-oriented research training:

> **Recommendation 4.4. The National Institute of Mental Health should support those departments that are poised to improve their residency-based research training to achieve measurable increases in patient-oriented research careers among their trainees. Support for such programs should include funds to:**
>
> - **Hire faculty and staff dedicated to research and research training efforts.**
> - **Acquire equipment and enhance facilities for research training.**
> - **Initiate pilot and/or short-term research activities for residents.**
> - **Educate adult and child and adolescent residency training directors and other faculty in how to promote and guide research career planning.**

Personal Factors

Individuals considering patient-oriented research in psychiatry are likely influenced by a number of personal factors. Some of these factors are so intrinsic that it is difficult to imagine the formal educational process, especially in adulthood, having a large impact on them. Perhaps the best any discipline can do with regard to candidates having exceptional drive or talent is to encourage them toward that specialty. There is some evidence that psychiatry may not be competitive in attracting the top or most research-intensive medical students (Feifel et al., 1999; Nicholson, 2002), despite unparalleled opportunities in the clinical brain and behavioral sciences. Part of the problem may be the compensation of psychiatrists as compared with that for other disciplines. The anticipated salaries for psychiatrists, whether academic or clinical, are near the bottom of the physician pay scale (AAMC, 2002b; Bureau of Labor Statistics, 2002). Concerns about loan repayment and overall financial well-being may discourage potential patient-oriented researchers from extended research training, which would further delay them from achieving their full earning potential. Although financial incentives for research experiences in core residency would create unacceptable compensation inequities, incentives for pursuing a research fellowship are limited only by the availability of funds. Accordingly, another recommendation the committee makes is as follows:

> **Recommendation 5.1. The National Institute of Mental Health and other funding agencies should seek mechanisms to offer increased financial incentives, such as loan repayment, to trainees who commit to research training and research involvement beyond core psychiatry residency.**

Although financial expectations play a role in the career decisions of medical students and residents, trainees are equally if not more concerned about other issues, such as lifestyle and the intellectual content of their selected profession. Furthermore, new physicians are understandably anxious about the challenges involved in securing long-term research funding and the workload associated with a research career. The committee observed that in recent years, many well-respected medical experts have written extensively about the problems associated with clinical research without promoting the endeavor as an exciting option for new physicians (Lieberman, 2001; Schrier, 1997; Shine, 1998). The preface to a recent opinion piece by an established psychiatrist-researcher, for example, notes that research careers are neither glamorous nor intellectually exciting, but instead are tedious and often involve considerable delayed gratification (Lieberman, 2001). While such characterizations are sometimes true of any difficult endeavor, the committee is concerned that they may overshadow the many positive aspects of a research career. Thus we make the following recommendation:

> **Recommendation 5.2. Individuals and institutions involved in the education and mentoring of medical students, residents and fellows should strongly convey to these trainees the benefits (professional and societal) associated with patient-oriented research in psychiatry. Promotion strategies might include support for student interest groups; brochures, websites, and other media; and summer research training opportunities.**

This recommendation is based on the belief that research offers a number of nonsalary benefits (e.g., a broad network of colleagues, involvement in new discoveries). This recommendation also encourages recruitment strategies that emphasize the growing scientific evidence base underlying the practice of modern psychiatry (Charney et al., 2001; Hamburg, 2002).

Finally, the demographics of the psychiatry workforce suggest that special measures are needed to ensure that talented women and international medical graduates are encouraged to pursue careers in patient-oriented research. Additionally, as is the case for all branches of medicine, greater involvement of underrepresented minorities is imperative if psychiatry is to offer the most responsive care to a diverse U.S. population. Accordingly, the committee makes the following three recommendations:

Recommendation 5.3. Departments of psychiatry, supported by the National Institute of Mental Health and other psychiatric organizations, should provide leadership in recruiting and retaining more women for psychiatry research careers. Such efforts should include:

- **Increasing part-time training and job sharing opportunities.**
- **Developing a critical mass of female role models and mentors.**
- **Working with institutions to improve child day care programs.**
- **Addressing institutional promotion and tenure issues, such as the tenure clock, that may be perceived as barriers to female trainees.**
- **Educating women about the time flexibility of research careers.**

Recommendation 5.4. Psychiatry training programs, academic medical centers, psychiatry organizations, and the federal government should work together to facilitate research training for international medical graduates who have the potential to make outstanding research contributions to psychiatry. Retention of the most productive of these international graduates in U.S. academic psychiatry programs should also be a joint effort.

Recommendation 5.5. Psychiatry research training programs should increase the numbers of underrepresented minority researchers by employing the following strategies:

- **Recruit minority faculty in multiple disciplines to serve as role models and mentors.**
- **Pursue funding from NIMH and other funding agencies that support minority trainees and faculty.**
- **Inform more minority psychiatrists about research training and other funding opportunities.**

Cross-Cutting Themes and Future Directions

Two points emerged from the committee's broad review of the problem of encouraging psychiatry residents to pursue careers in research. First, numerous factors influence a psychiatry resident's decision about a research career. Second, despite numerous national and local efforts, there is a paucity of data about which methods are truly effective at fostering research career development and success among psychiatrists. Accordingly, the recommendations of this report are based in large part upon the expert opinions of the committee members.

Regarding the first point, there is a fairly extensive body of opinion and anecdotal evidence to support the relevance of each of the regulatory, institutional, and personal factors summarized above. Detailed analyses of the factors impacting research training are quite rare, however, and the committee is aware of very few studies that attempt to quantify the relative contribution of specific variables (Kruse et al., 2003; Pincus et al., 1995). As an example of the uncertainty that remains, it is currently impossible to determine whether spending more on mentors or on enhancing trainee recruitment would yield greater gains in the numbers of patient-oriented researchers in psychiatry.

Most of the committee's recommendations are likely relevant to physician-investigators outside of psychiatry. However, issues of stigma and the history of the profession weigh more heavily for psychiatry than for other medical specialties with regard to research and research training (DHHS, 1999; Eisenberg, 2002). Additionally, a theme of this report is that what is true for adult psychiatry is even more so for child and adolescent psychiatry. Specifically, there appears to be a particular shortage of child and adolescent psychiatrists and psychiatrist-researchers despite the many challenges posed by mental disorders affecting the nation's youth (Kim et al., 2001).

Finally, the committee found that data regarding (1) the need for psychiatrist researchers and (2) the success and precise strategies of individual programs that purport to train them, were both lacking despite strong interest and action by numerous stakeholders. Although there is evidence supporting the hypothesis that an increase in psychiatrist-researchers would benefit the nation's mental health, this contention has not been well substantiated in a systematic and scientific way. Similarly, while there are many isolated efforts to train psychiatrist researchers, there is at best implicit coordination between some of these efforts suggesting that increase cooperation may yield benefits to the psychiatric research workforce more broadly. Better data on the numbers of psychiatrist-researchers and their contribution to the nation's mental health will likely be necessary to convince policy makers and medical educators that the training of psychiatrist-researchers is worthy of increased investment. Given this need for more information, and the need to insure coordination among various groups engaged in research training, the committee makes the following overarching recommendation:

> **Recommendation 6.1. The National Institute of Mental Health should take the lead in organizing a national body, including major stakeholders (e.g., patient groups, department chairs) and representatives of organizations in psychiatry, that will foster the integration of research into psychiatric residency and monitor outcomes of efforts to do so. This group should specifically collect and analyze relevant data, develop strategies to be put into practice, and measure the effectiveness of existing and novel approaches aimed at training patient-oriented researchers in psychiatry. The group should have direct consultative authority with the director of the National Institute of Mental Health, and also should provide concise periodic reports to all interested stakeholders regarding its accomplishments and future goals.**

Many national organizations, including the American Psychiatric Association and the American Academy of Child and Adolescent Psychiatry, are already directly addressing the problem of research training in psychiatry. This recommendation aims to encourage maximal cooperation among these organizations so that redundancy is avoided, and systematic and large-scale assessments of best practices can be undertaken. The recommendation is also intended to bring together stakeholders in psychiatry and related disciplines to pursue the goal of defining more precisely the specific contributions psychiatrists can and have made to biomedical research.

Table ES-1 summarizes the committee's recommendations and identifies the obstacles to research training in psychiatric residency addressed by each.

EXECUTIVE SUMMARY

TABLE ES-1 Summary of Recommendations

Topic	Number	Recommendation	Obstacle Addressed
Longitudinal Perspective	2.1	Foster coordinated multiyear research training experiences.	Research opportunities are fragmented across the multiple levels and years of training.
Regulatory Factors	3.1	Increase the flexibility of training requirements.	Clinical requirements are excessive and prevent tailored training.
	3.2	Require research literacy.	Many training programs lack research education components.
	3.3	Require researcher membership on regulatory bodies.	Researchers are not sufficiently involved in setting expectations for training curricula and achievement of competencies.
Institutional Factors	4.1	Encourage executives to invest in mental health research.	Resources to support research training are limited; stigma works against optimal mental health care funding.
	4.2	Encourage research faculty involvement.	Researchers often are not involved in direct resident training.
	4.3	Create patient-oriented research training curricula.	Curricula are needed that incorporate research training across the range and time constraints of residency programs.
	4.4	Support emerging programs.	Resources to move programs to the next level of research training are scarce.
Personal Factors	5.1	Increase financial compensation to trainees.	Education debt and low compensation deter the choice of a research career.
	5.2	Develop strategies to attract trainees to patient-oriented research.	Trainees have pessimistic views of research careers and can be uninformed about research opportunities.
	5.3	Develop women researchers.	Talent is underutilized.
	5.4	Develop international medical graduate researchers.	Talent is underutilized.
	5.5	Develop minority researchers.	Workforce diversity is lacking; talent is underutilized.
Overarching Recommendation	6.1	Establish a national coordinating effort.	Monitoring data are lacking, and there is no centralized plan for research training.

1

Introduction

STUDY CONTEXT

The Burden of Mental Illness

Recent global estimates suggest that at any one time, 450 million persons suffer from neuropsychiatric disorders, including depression and/or mania, schizophrenia, epilepsy, alcohol and other addictive disorders, dementias, anxiety disorders, and serious sleep disturbances (World Health Organization [WHO], 2001). In terms of disability-adjusted life years, a measure that combines estimates of disease morbidity and mortality, mental disease ranks second only to cardiovascular disorders, and first if one includes the burden of suicide and substance abuse. Specifically, 1991 data coalesced by WHO, Harvard University, and others indicate that 15.4 percent of the total disease burden in industrialized countries can be directly attributed to mental disorders.[2] By comparison, only cardiovascular diseases rank higher, at 18.6 percent. Cancer is a close third, at 15 percent, while respiratory diseases (6.2 percent) and alcohol-related morbidity (4.7 percent) are a distant fourth and fifth, respectively (U.S. Department of Health and Human Services [DHHS], 1999; Murray and Lopez, 1996).

Millions of Americans experience the debilitating and sometimes deadly consequences of mental illness: 10 million suffer from a major depressive disorder (National Institute of Mental Health [NIMH], 2001c), over 2 million adults suffer from schizophrenia (Hoyert et al., 1999), and 30,000 individuals commit suicide each year (NIMH, 2001c). Serious mental disorders also afflict a large number of children. Severe or extreme functional impairment related to such diseases (e.g., depression, anorexia nervosa, violent behaviors, and autistic-spectrum abnor-

---

[2] Mental disorders include unipolar major depression, schizophrenia, bipolar disorder, obsessive-compulsive disorder, panic disorder, post-traumatic stress disorder, and self-inflicted injuries (e.g., suicide). Excluded are substance-abuse disorders that include alcohol addiction.

malities) is estimated to occur in 4 to 10 percent of individuals under the age of 18 (Friedman et al., 1996; Kim et al., 2001; Leebens et al., 1993). Diagnosable mental illness of all severities is believed to exist in 12 to 24 percent of school-aged children (Foa et al., 2000; Friedman et al., 1996; Kim et al., 2001; Shaffer et al., 1996).

Increasing Societal Awareness of Mental Illness

In response to such mental health problems, and given the promise of brain and behavioral research to address these problems, the 1990s was officially dubbed the "the decade of the brain," and entry into the new millennium has been assigned a complementary label, "the decade of behavior" (Decade of Behavior, 2001; Library of Congress, 2000). Between 1999 and 2002, the U.S. Surgeon General released several reports focused on mental health, including two broad-ranging reports on the subject (one general and one focused on ethnic, cultural, and racial issues), as well as reports on tobacco addiction and on youth violence (DHHS, 2001a; 2001b; 2001c; 2002). In 2001, WHO also released a comprehensive report on the state of global mental health (WHO, 2001). In 2002, a White House Commission on the U.S. mental health care delivery system released its interim report (President's New Freedom Commission on Mental Health, 2002).

All of the above reports detail the extraordinary gains that have been made in mental health care, including advances in integrative neuroscience and health services research. Yet they also point to substantial gaps in basic and clinical scientific knowledge related to the treatment and prevention of mental diseases, gaps that must be filled by the efforts of a sophisticated workforce consisting of physicians, epidemiologists, psychologists, and neuroscientists. Collectively, these reports reflect the unambiguous emergence of mental health care as a key priority in the United States and internationally.

Advances in Mental Health Care

Substantial and increasing public awareness and activity regarding brain function and disease have evolved along with impressive research progress in the neural and behavioral sciences. Numerous innovations and discoveries can be cited that enhance our understanding of the human brain and the delivery of care to those who suffer from mental disorders. Genetic and other molecular research has exposed elements of the biological underpinnings of several severe behavioral disorders, including depression, schizophrenia, dementia, and substance abuse (e.g., Charney et al., 2001; Hyman, 2002a). Neuroimaging advances have permitted noninvasive, in vivo views of brain anatomy, metabolism, and dynamic function (Bertolino and Weinberger, 1999; Durston et al., 2001; Fu and McGuire, 1999; Hendren et al., 2000; Malhi et al., 2002; Marder and May, 1986; Moresco et al., 2001; Royall et al., 2002; Yanai, 1999). Pharmacologic and psychologic therapies, alone or in combination, have demonstrated considerable efficacy in treating a variety of mental disorders, including schizophrenia, dementia, depression, anxiety and panic disorders, obsessive-compulsive disorder, hyperactivity, inattention, post-traumatic stress disorder, and substance abuse (Barton, 2000; Beck, 1993; Borkovec and Ruscio, 2001; Chambless and Ollendick, 2001; Kane et al., 1988; Klerman, 1989; Lambert, 2001; Leon, 1979; Lewinsohn et al., 1998; Marder and May, 1986; Nathan and Gorman, 1998; President's New Freedom Commission on Mental Health, 2002; Schou, 1997; Shaffer et al., 1996; Trinh et al., 2003; Weston and Morrison, 2001). And health services research investigations have identified correlates to cost-effective and high-quality psychiatric care (Corsico and McGuffin, 2001; Schoenbaum et al., 2001).

Accordingly, the current situation can be summarized as follows. Great advances have been made in mental health care in recent years, and technological advances in the basic and clinical neural and behavioral sciences offer considerable promise for future gains. At the same time, the burden of mental illness remains very high, perhaps higher than that of any other single category of disease. Public knowledge about mental illness is increasing, as is public support for continued research. These realities should logically coincide with the growing involvement of psychiatrists in patient-oriented research.

Psychiatrists are in a good position to answer relevant etiologic, preventive, and treatment questions about mental illness because they are trained in the biological and psychological basis of such illness, and because they have extensive experience in observing and treating the complexities of a wide variety of moderate to severe behavioral and emotional disorders. The importance of researchers with credentials in psychiatry is predicated on the logic that they have a valuable and unique set of skills and perspectives encompassing the clinical neurosciences, psychopharmacology, psychotherapy, mental illness diagnostics, and integrative human physiology (Andreasen, 2001). These skills place psychiatrists trained in research methods in an excellent position to assess the broad clinical needs of individuals with mental disorders and to frame questions that are relevant to improving patient care. Accordingly, while a neuroscientist might offer critical information about the importance of a specific neurotransmitter in the pathophysiology that underlies a given brain disease, and a clinical psychologist might effectively measure the associated behavioral symptoms or deliver psychotherapy, it may well be that a psychiatrist is needed to bridge these sophisticated elements to enable the design of a safe and clinically relevant experiment that can yield meaningful insights regarding a novel therapy. For all of these reasons and certainly others, psychiatrists occupy an important and unique niche in the spectrum of neuroscientists and behavioral scientists, and increasing the ranks of psychiatrist-researchers as principal and co-investigators would, in the view of the committee, accelerate advances in mental health.

As more objective evidence that psychiatrists contribute to the research enterprise, a recent assessment of published and peer-reviewed literature found that from 1990 to 1998, 16 of the top 22 cited authors of psychiatry articles had been trained as psychiatrists. Included in that assessment were at least 16 of the most reputed psychiatry journals (e.g., *Archives of General Psychiatry, British Journal of Psychiatry, Journal of the American Academy of Child and Adolescent Psychiatry*) and the multidisciplinary journals *Science, Nature,* and *Proceedings of the National Academy of Sciences*. Authors were ranked only if they had published at least 15 high-impact papers during that 8-year period, high-impact being defined as those among the 200 most cited papers during a given year. The most cited psychiatry article during that period was coauthored by a psychiatrist and a non-psychiatrist: Ronald C. Kessler, a sociologist at the University of Michigan,[3] and Kenneth S. Kendler, a psychiatrist at Virginia Commonwealth University. These two authors published "Lifetime and 12-month prevalence of DSM-III-R psychiatric disorders in the United States: Results from the National Comorbidity Survey" in 1994, in addition to more than 30 other high-impact papers during the 8-year period assessed (ISI Thomson, 2003). Their most cited paper is clearly patient-oriented as it reports on empirically-derived epidemiologic information regarding a number of mental disorders. It also demonstrates the potential productivity that can result from collaborations between psychiatrists and Ph.D. investigators.

---

[3] Currently Professor in the Department of Health Care Policy, Harvard Medical School.

GENESIS OF THE STUDY

Trends in Training of Psychiatrist-Researchers

NIMH is at the center of U.S. efforts to safeguard mental health and is, accordingly, a principal source of funding for psychiatrist trainees and established researchers. In 2001, NIMH provided more than $230 million in training and research grants to psychiatrist-investigators, and since 1987, well over 60 percent of all extramural grant funding from this institute has gone to either psychiatrist (27–33 percent) or psychologist (36–41 percent) principal investigators (data courtesy of NIMH, Office of Science Policy and Program Policy, February 21, 2003). It is therefore cause for considerable concern that NIMH officials, along with other prominent leaders in psychiatry, believe the training of psychiatrist-researchers is not keeping pace with needs in patient-oriented mental health research (Fenton, 2002; Hyman, 2001; 2002b; Hyman and Fenton, 2003; Kupfer et al., 2002; Shore et al., 2001). This concern stems from data indicating a general decline in physician-researchers across medicine (Ahrens, 1992; Institute of Medicine [IOM], 1994; NIH, 1997b; National Research Council [NRC], 2000; Rosenberg, 2000; Schrier, 1997; Shine, 1998; Wyngaarden, 1979; Zemlo et al., 2000). Data on psychiatrists per se support that contention, although it is not altogether clear whether the numbers of psychiatrist-researchers are declining or simply stagnating at a time when mental health issues have come to the forefront of health concerns in the United States (as discussed above). The extent to which psychiatrist-researchers are needed is also unclear, given that psychologists and other Ph.D. investigators conduct a large and valuable proportion of psychiatric research. Nevertheless, the position of psychiatry appears to be particularly weak with regard to research, and there are data to support that contention.

Between 1992 and 2002, the entire NIH budget increased by 55 percent in current dollars, as did the budgets for NIMH and the National Institutes of Neurological Disorders and Stroke (NINDS), Drug Abuse (NIDA), and Alcohol Abuse and Alcoholism (NIAAA)—the four principal institutes that focus on diseases of the brain and behavior. During this same period, the numbers of NIMH-funded psychiatrists as principal investigators kept reasonable pace (see Figure 1-1), although there certainly has been no increase in the relative proportion of psychiatrists in the principal investigator role. If anything there has been a slight decrease, from 33 percent to 27 percent of principal investigators. Similarly, broad surveys of U.S. physicians conducted annually by the

American Medical Association (AMA) indicate that since 1988, the proportion of practicing psychiatrists claiming research as their predominant activity has hovered close to a mere 2 percent (data courtesy of the Association of American Medical Colleges [AAMC], Section for Institutional and Faculty Studies, July 2003). The fact that only 2 percent of practicing psychiatrists spend more than 50 percent of their time engaged in research compares poorly with analogous research involvement rates for several other disciplines of medicine (see Table 1-1), disciplines that are themselves experiencing declining numbers of physician-investigators (Ahrens, 1992; Zemlo et al., 2000).

Other direct sources of data on the number of psychiatrist-researchers were difficult to obtain, but at least two sources support the conclusion that research involvement among practicing psychiatrists in the United States and Canada is exceedingly low. Pincus et al. (1993) used 1989 data, collected through a self-report survey, indicating that within academic departments of psychiatry at accredited medical schools, 25.8 percent of non–Ph.D.-holding M.D.'s spent at least 1 day per week engaged in some form of research. For internal medicine, the

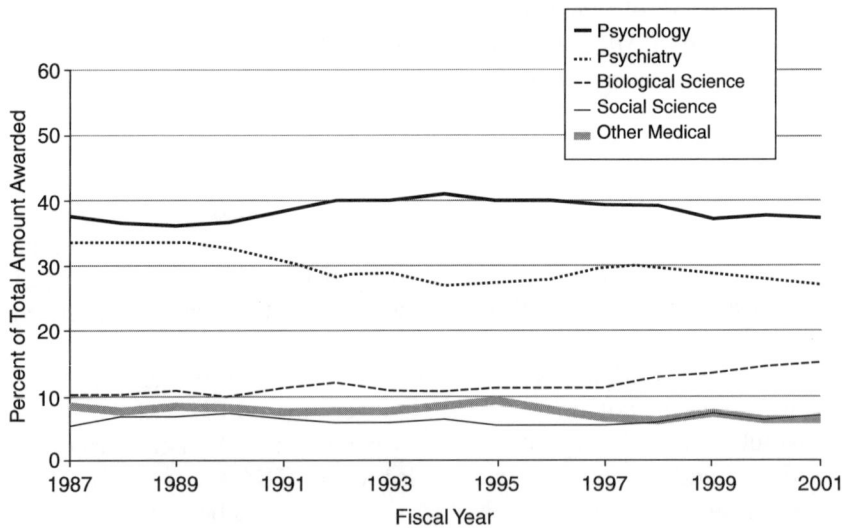

FIGURE 1-1 Percent of National Institute of Mental Health (NIMH) extramural grants (including research, fellowship, and institutional training grants) stratified by the five major disciplines of the corresponding principal investigators.
SOURCE: Data courtesy of NIMH, Office of Science Policy and Program Policy, February 21, 2003.

TABLE 1-1 Research Involvement Rates of Practicing Psychiatrists and Other Selected M.D. Specialists, Years 1999 and 2000

Discipline	Research Rate[a] in 2000 (percent)	Research Rate[a] in 1999 (percent)	Number of Active Physicians in 2000	Number Citing Research as Primary Activity in 2000	Number of Active Physicians in 1999	Number Citing Research as Primary Activity in 1999
Psychiatry	2.0	1.9	45,737	913	44,935	870
Neurology	6.3	6.4	12,357	773	11,638	744
Internal Medicine Subspecialties[b]	6.1	6.1	87,114	5,327	85,672	5,264

NOTE: Rates are the proportion of all psychiatrists declaring research as their primary professional activity.
[a]Research rate = (number of survey respondents citing research as primary activity)/(number of active physicians).
[b]Aggregates numbers from the following specialties: allergy and immunology, cardiovascular diseases, dermatology, gastroenterology, internal medicine (other, not general), and pulmonary diseases.
SOURCE: Pasko and Seidman (2002), AAMC (2002b).

relative proportion of researchers among M.D.'s was nearly twice that, at 41.9 percent. Using more recent data from a 1998 national sample of psychiatrists both within and outside of academic departments of psychiatry, Schwalm (2002a) found that 19.8 percent of responding psychiatrists report some involvement in research (see Chapter 5). Given that this rate of 19.8 includes psychiatrists who spend as little as 1 percent of their time on research, it is logically an overestimate of the proportion of psychiatrists who engage in a meaningful level of research.[4] Although these two separate data sources cannot be used to characterize a decline over time, they do indicate that research involvement for psychiatrists have been and continue to be very low. These sources reveal unequivocally that at best only about one in five practicing psychiatrists engages in any research activity, and that if the figures are the same as they were in 1989, only about one in four psychiatrists at U.S. medical schools spends more than 1 day a week adding to the knowledge base of the profession.

Finally, and perhaps most disturbing, research training in psychiatry may be on the decline, as indicated by recent surveys of advertised research fellowships for psychiatrists. Fellowships are training periods that typically occur immediately after residency. The American Psychiatric Association (APA) compiles annual lists of research fellowship opportunities for physicians who have just completed their psychiatric residency training. This survey represents a conscientious and high-profile[5] attempt by the APA to include all of the research training programs in the United States and Canada at accredited allopathic medical schools—the most logical venues for physician research training programs. Results from the 1992, 1995, and 2001 surveys indicate declines in every category related to research training, including the numbers of institutions, training programs, and M.D.-trained fellows engaged in that training. For example, in 1992 there were 282 M.D.'s recorded in the APA fellowship compilation; in 1995 the number had dropped to 239; and as of 2001 it was at 178 (Guerra and Regier, 2001; Nevin and Pincus, 1992; Steele and Pincus, 1995). Although this survey was not designed as a quantitative assessment of the number of research trainees, the steady decline in their numbers is especially striking, and if it truly reflects a contraction of such programs, it is likely that even fewer new psychiatrists will be pre-

---

[4] Additional analyses provided by Schwalm indicate that less than 3 percent of practicing psychiatrists spend more than 30 percent of their professional time engaged in research.

[5] The APA is the largest professional society for psychiatrists in the United States. The most recent version of the survey involved as many as four separate mailings to department chairs and program directors to encourage their response. The APA uses the data collected to promote all the programs by publishing a guide for prospective fellows.

pared for substantive research careers over the next several years (Fenton, 2002).

With the above trends in mind, NIMH asked the IOM to conduct a study aimed at determining what factors influence psychiatric residents to consider research careers.

Study Charge

Given the unparalleled opportunities and needs that exist in mental health research and the apparent decline in the number of psychiatrists entering the research workforce, NIMH commissioned the IOM to address the following four tasks:

1. Review the goals and objectives of training for adult and child psychiatry residents with an emphasis on both core research training and training trajectories to facilitate patient-oriented research career development. This review would provide advice to the Accreditation Council for Graduate Medical Education (ACGME), Residency Review Committee (RRC), and psychiatry community prior to the next cycle of revising residency requirements.

2. Review the experiences of psychiatry residency programs that currently incorporate research and succeed in training successful patient-oriented adult and child psychiatrist researchers. Assess the strategies these programs use and their applicability to other training programs, especially non-research oriented programs. Define new strategies to allow research-training opportunities for psychiatry residents in less research-intensive training settings.

3. Determine obstacles to offering research opportunities to psychiatry residents. These may include access to role models and mentors, economic concerns, and impact of existing training requirements. Consider approaches to overcome these obstacles.

4. Provide strategies for psychiatry residency training that permit research experience and/or more intensive research training tracks while meeting the re-

quirements for clinical competency in adult and child psychiatry.

Composition of the Committee

To respond to the above charge, the IOM appointed a committee of 12 members broadly representing psychiatry (both adult and child and adolescent from small and large programs), other biological and cognitive–behavioral disciplines (neurology, psychology, neuroscience), mental health economics, and other branches of medicine (pathology and pediatrics). Committee members either were experienced in training biomedical researchers or had direct experience in the field of graduate medical education. The committee included two psychiatry department chairs, a medical school dean, and a director of a children's hospital research foundation.

STUDY APPROACH AND SCOPE

Overall Strategy

The committee's work extended over a 16-month period commencing in March 2002. During that period, the committee held five 2-day meetings that included both closed-session deliberations and open sessions for dialogue with experts and stakeholders. The second committee meeting coincided with a full-day public workshop focused on obstacles to research training during psychiatric residency. The committee also gathered information through numerous personal contacts, two commissioned papers, outreach mailings to members of the American Association of Directors of Psychiatric Residency Training, literature reviews, and Internet searches. Appendix A offers additional detail on the study sources and methods.

Definitions and Broad Concepts

From its deliberations, discussions with NIMH officials, and other sources, the committee formulated the following definitions and concepts that are utilized throughout this report.

INTRODUCTION

Residency as the Focus: One Point on a Continuum

Residency is a program of study and clinical training lasting 3 or more years that follows graduation from medical school and precedes certification in a given medical specialty (e.g., psychiatry). *Fellowship*, by contrast, is 1 or more years of additional training that follows residency. Fellowships usually result in additional certification and/or subspecialization (e.g., addiction psychiatry, research). The study charge directed the committee to study the residency and training trajectories relevant to research career development. The committee believes these trajectories encompass experiences in close proximity to residency training, including those before (e.g., medical school) and after (e.g., fellowship and junior faculty) residency. One notable limitation of this aspect of the study charge is that it does not include later career phases, when previously productive researchers may leave the field because of a lack of funding or a desire to pursue other professional interests and responsibilities (Pincus, 2001b). Nevertheless, the committee believes that evaluation of early career training is a reasonable starting point from which to assess research activity by psychiatrists more broadly.

Adult Psychiatry, Subspecialists, and Nonpsychiatrists

The study charge directed the committee to consider specifically both adult and child psychiatry residencies. Technically, *adult psychiatry* residents are nonentities as all psychiatry residents receive marginal child and adolescent training,[6] thereby affording them the designation of *general psychiatrists*. Furthermore, this so-called general training is the foundation upon which other psychiatric training, including the two-year child and adolescent fellowship training, is currently built (Accreditation Council for Graduate Medical Education [ACGME], 2000b). This contrasts child psychiatry training to pediatrics training as the latter is independent from its logical adult-centered counterpart, internal medicine. Accordingly, for simplicity and in keeping with the charge, general psychiatry will heretofore be referred to as adult psychiatry and the child and adolescent fellowship that immediately follows general training will be referred to as a residency.

Child psychiatry likely received explicit mention in the study charge because there is broad consensus among mental health professionals that

---

[6] Only 2 months of the 36-month training program in general psychiatry is dedicated to child and adolescent psychiatry.

there is a severe shortage of experts trained to care for children and adolescents with mental disorders (DHHS, 1999; 2000; Kim et al., 2001). Data from NIMH offer some indication of how that shortage may be influencing research participation by child psychiatrists. Although there are seven adult psychiatrists for every child psychiatrist, data from NIMH indicate that from 1993 to 2001, the number of principal investigators in psychiatry favored adult psychiatrist-researchers by a ratio of 11 to 1. Similarly in 2001, of $130 million in R01 grant[7] dollars paid to all psychiatrist–principal investigators, only $14 million (less than 11 percent) was paid to child and adolescent psychiatrists.[8] The especially low numbers for child psychiatrist–researchers thus support their special consideration in this report on research training.

Although this report emphasizes broad psychiatric training by focusing on both adult and child and adolescent training, this emphasis is not intended to minimize the importance of patient-oriented research training for psychiatric subspecialists not explicitly noted in the study charge (i.e., geriatrics, addiction, forensics, pain management). Similarly, this focus is not meant to downplay the psychiatric research contributions and training needs of social and life scientists in other disciplines (e.g., psychologists, neuroscientists) (IOM, 2000). The involvement of psychologists in patient-oriented psychiatric research is, in fact, an important component of psychiatry. Data presented to the committee by Roger Meyer of the Association of American Medical Colleges showed that psychiatry departments are second only to internal medicine departments with regard to their aggregate research budgets (Meyer, 2002; NIH, 2003b). However, it is also the case that well over half of that funding (59 percent) appears to be attributable to the efforts of Ph.D. investigators, whereas in internal medicine and neurology departments, Ph.D.'s make up less than 33 percent of the NIH-funded researchers (Fang and Meyer, 2003).

This discrepancy in dependence on Ph.D. research capacity likely is related to the fact that psychology and psychiatry have a uniquely large proportion of intellectual and practical overlap as compared with other academic physicians and their Ph.D. colleagues. The discrepancy also raises the question of whether low numbers of psychiatrist-researchers may be functionally offset by the presence of many capable Ph.D.-credentialed researchers. On the one hand, it is the case that Ph.D.-

---

[7] R01 grants are the most common grant mechanism used by the National Institutes of Health to fund extramural researchers.

[8] Raw data courtesy of the NIMH, Office of Science Policy and Program Policy, February 21, 2003. Analysis done by IOM staff.

trained researchers, especially psychologists, play a substantive role in psychiatric patient-oriented research. On the other hand, it is the committee's belief that psychiatrists bring a unique perspective to that endeavor as trained physicians in the clinical brain and behavior sciences. Accordingly, though not well validated by any hard data, the committee's opinion is that the study charge is reasonable in its aim to incrementally increase the level of psychiatrist-researchers. Finally, although this goal may appear to favor a "guild" within mental health, its focus on psychiatrists need not represent a "zero sum game" in which having more psychiatrist-researchers corresponds to having fewer psychologists or neuroscientists engaged in that endeavor. Instead, the focus on psychiatrists is aimed at careful analysis of the state of one readily definable sector of the mental health workforce.

Patient-Oriented Research

According to a 1999 NIH program announcement, *patient-oriented research* is "...conducted with human subjects (or on material of human origin such as tissues, specimens, and cognitive phenomena) for which an investigator directly interacts with human subjects. This area of research includes: (1) mechanisms of human disease; (2) therapeutic interventions; (3) clinical trials; and (4) the development of new technologies" (NIH, 1999b). Accordingly, the definition is fairly broad and overlaps with that of *clinical research*, although clinical research does not necessarily require patient interaction. Patient-oriented research also overlaps with *translational research*, which aims to translate "bench" or more basic research advances into technologies that reduce human suffering from disease. Patient-oriented research does not include basic research that is designed to elucidate the details of normal human or animal physiology. The definition is otherwise fairly broad and includes such efforts as health services research, outcomes research, molecular studies, and epidemiologic studies, as long as they include some data collection directly from human subjects (AAMC, 1999; Association for Patient Oriented Research, 2000; IOM, 1994; Meyer et al., 1998; NIAAA, 2002; National Institute of Child Health and Development [NICHD], 2002; NIH, 1997a; 1997b; NIMH, 2000b).

Limitations of the Data

Given that the general problem of the "endangered" physician-investigator emerged nearly 25 years ago (Wyngaarden, 1979), considerable data are available regarding the aggregate of physician-investigators (IOM, 1994; Zemlo et al., 2000); data on subspecialties are more difficult to come by, however. NIMH, for example, provided the committee with some data stratifying the institute's extramural investigator portfolio by specialty (e.g., psychologist, adult [general] and child and adolescent psychiatrists), but such stratification appears to be new, and thus these data have yet to be carefully scrutinized. Likewise, data on research training approaches are limited in medicine generally and in psychiatry in particular. Accordingly, the committee rarely found well-designed studies in which one group that received a certain type of research training or other exposure was compared with a group that did not. The committee also found that most programs do not carefully track their graduates to determine whether they are researchers, let alone whether they are clinical researchers and to what extent they are engaged and productive in that endeavor. More common in the research training literature and department record keeping is a method of "creaming" for outcome data—that is, describing the success stories and ignoring or downplaying the failures. Such descriptions are used throughout this report and are useful in the face of little other information. Thus, the committee acknowledges that this report is based in large part on its expert judgment, and reliant upon much qualitative and often incomplete data from outside contributors. One important future need identified in this report is for additional tracking and assessment of research training outcomes.

ORGANIZATION OF THE REPORT

The remainder of this report is organized into five chapters. **Chapter 2** develops a rationale for residency as a target of patient-oriented research training. In that chapter, residency is placed in the context of a broader career continuum that includes medical school and fellowship training. The chapter begins by describing the benefits of incorporating research training into residency. It then addresses the importance of linking research training in residency to research exposures before (e.g., medical school) and after (e.g., fellowship) that time. The chapter concludes with some general themes regarding long-term training and a brief description of training models outside of psychiatry.

Chapters 3 through **5** address in turn the following three major sets of factors that influence research training: *regulatory*, *institutional*, and *personal*.

More specifically, **Chapter 3** reviews regulatory issues and, per item 1 of the committee's charge, is focused in particular on the Residency Review Committee program requirements for psychiatry and other residencies, which must be met by all programs wishing to be accredited to train medical specialists, including psychiatrists. This chapter also briefly describes the role of the American Board of Psychiatry and Neurology and several other organizations and professional societies with regard to residency-based research training.

Chapter 4 examines institutional issues related to research training within a department of psychiatry and more broadly within the individual hospitals or universities. The chapter begins by describing the idiosyncrasies and challenges associated with the funding of graduate medical education, and then turns to leadership and mentoring issues. The chapter concludes with a review of local and national program strategies (e.g., curricula) currently being used to train clinical researchers within and outside of psychiatry.

Chapter 5 moves from the extrinsic factors reviewed in Chapters 3 and 4 to the more intrinsic or personal factors that influence research training in the context of the psychiatric residency. Motivation and intellectual capacity are briefly discussed as a reminder that certain factors transcend programmatic structure or resources. Personal finances, including debt and training stipends, are also addressed in this chapter. Finally, issues of race and gender are discussed, as are the unique issues faced by foreign medical school graduates.

At the close of Chapters 2 through 5, the committee offers recommendations corresponding to the respective topics. A final **Chapter 6** offers some future directions for action beyond the recommendations cast in Chapters 2 through 5. That chapter also addresses the need for better data to characterize the psychiatrist-researcher workforce and the effectiveness of individual and national training programs.

The report ends with four appendices. Appendix A describes the methods used for this study and the open-session meetings and public workshops hosted by the committee. Appendix B lists funding opportunities for individuals and programs interested in developing their research training portfolios. Appendix C provides brief programmatic characteristics of selected residency training programs. Finally, Appendix D contains biographical sketches of committee members and study staff.

2

Residency as Part of a Longitudinal Career Continuum

The previous chapter detailed the need for and apparent shortfall in the number of psychiatrist-researchers. This chapter places residency in the broad longitudinal continuum of physician training, ranging from the undergraduate years, to medical school, residency, fellowship, and beyond. It begins by examining why residency is a critical juncture for career planning and at least some research training. It then describes the importance of research training and exposure before and after residency, as well as how such training and exposure are implemented in psychiatry, internal medicine, and pediatrics. Strategic considerations involved in providing an integrated, longitudinal research experience are addressed, and brief descriptions of existing mechanisms for serving this purpose are presented. The chapter ends with conclusions and a single recommendation regarding longitudinal research training associated with residency.

RESIDENCY AS AN IMPORTANT TARGET FOR RESEARCH TRAINING

Residency is the last obligatory stage of preprofessional education for most psychiatrists (see Figure 2-1). Therefore, career differentiation occurs for many psychiatrists during this experience, which can be considered an essential node that connects medical school to one of several possible long-term career paths. Thus it makes sense to examine activities and other influences within residency that encourage or inhibit research career tracking.

The rationale for focusing on research training during residency must be clearly stated to justify the allocation of resources (e.g., time, funding) needed to increase residency research options. Several logical arguments are advanced below and are summarized in Box 2-1.

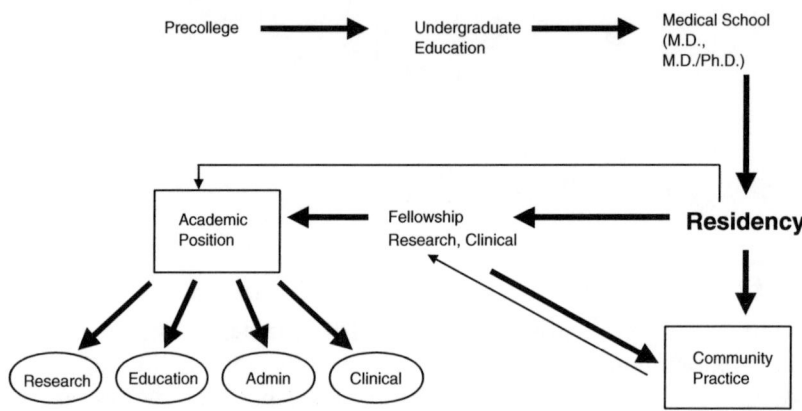

FIGURE 2-1 Training pathways in psychiatry.

BOX 2-1
Rationale for Incorporating Research Training into the Residency Experience

- Promotes research literacy for all trainees.
- Encourages future participation of clinicians as research collaborators.
- Provides experiences that may foster choosing a research career.
- Couples expanding clinical knowledge with the formulation of patient-oriented research questions.
- Attracts the curious and/or motivates medical students to psychiatry training.
- Maintains and furthers research interest among residents with investigative backgrounds.

Research Literacy

Research didactic learning or practical experiences in residency have the potential to promote research literacy—the ability to assimilate emerging theoretical knowledge about biology and empirical information relevant to a given set of symptoms and corresponding risk factors or treatments. Being research literate also means having the knowledge and ability to understand and convey to peers and patients the challenges that exist to the development of new knowledge. Accordingly, the ability to read the literature critically is important, as is an appreciation for the difficulty of creating, implementing, and interpreting an experimental protocol.

Stated another way, research literacy can be considered a prerequisite for the lifelong practice of evidence-based medicine that involves "explicit and judicious use of current best evidence" to care for patients (Sackett et al., 1996:71). Findings of surveys of psychiatry trainees and faculty appear to validate the notion that integration of research into residency enhances residents' ability to care for patients (Fitz-Gerald et al., 2001). Research literacy is particularly important given the quantity and variety of medical information that is routinely published and presented (Mulrow and Lohr, 2001). Moreover, research literacy may encourage research collaboration on the part of those who will spend a majority of their professional time in clinical care, providing clinical psychiatrists with the skills needed to serve knowledgeably as coinvestigators for research studies focused on psychiatric disease or for studies in which psychiatric comorbidity is important to overall patient health (e.g., depression in cancer patients). For example, increased appreciation of research may eliminate some of the barriers to subject recruitment that can result from misunderstanding of research protocols on the part of physicians or patients. Well-informed clinicians can help potential research subjects understand the limitations of a given research protocol, including the interpretation and practical use of clinical data that result from participation in the research. The concept of and need for a randomized and double-blind design may otherwise be unclear, even antithetical, to many patients. Research literate physicians also will be more equipped to characterize the uncertainties (e.g., probability, relative risk) of disease course or treatment outcomes to patients, and to do so using information that is constantly being updated by the latest technologies and scientific findings.

In summary, although much of medicine, including psychiatry, has a considerable evidence base supporting practice methods, the committee's strong sense is that residency-based exposure to research theory and practice can have a very positive effect on strengthening the evolution and implementation of the best psychiatric practices. Additionally, and most germane to this report, such exposure should encourage more psychiatrists to devote at least a portion of their professional training and time to research.

Exposures and Experiences

As suggested above, residency is a time of critical career decision making. If too few psychiatry trainees opt for research-intensive careers, the reasons may lie, at least in part, within the residency experience (Appelbaum et al., 1978; DeHaven et al., 1998). Exposure to research theory and practice in residency has not been assessed as frequently as such training in the context of postresidency fellowship, but there is some evidence that residency-based research training is an antecedent to future research career tracking, albeit from other disciplines. For example, a recent survey of 96 surgical residency graduates from the University of California at Los Angeles (a 65 percent response rate) demonstrated that those with at least 2 years of residency-based research laboratory experience were twice as likely as those with less training to track to an academic position (Dunn et al., 1998). DeHaven and colleagues (1998) conducted a broad telephone survey (n = 321) of family medicine residency programs (a 75 percent response rate), followed by a more targeted survey (n = 72) of recent graduates and training directors and in-depth interviews with 28 of the most research-intensive residency programs. They found that interest in practice-based research coincided with training programs in which a majority of residents had completed a research project, and in which there were opportunities for research that included program director support and a research curriculum.

Correlative studies examining the impact of fellowship training have been conducted in psychiatry as well as in other medical specialties (Davis and Kelley, 1982; Dial et al., 1990; Dunn et al., 1998; Haviland et al., 1987; Pincus et al., 1993; Ringel et al., 2001). Pincus and colleagues (1995) conducted a survey of 1,917 M.D. faculty members in departments of psychiatry from 116 U.S. medical schools. Using a fairly precise and inclusive definition of a "researcher" (i.e., only 20 percent of one's time engaged in research activities), they found that M.D.'s with postdoctoral research training were 4 times more likely to be researchers than their colleagues without such additional training. Lee and colleagues (1991) surveyed 2,642 clinical researchers (2,487 with MD degrees) and found that 1,371 of them had received federal research funding. Multivariate analysis further found that research training during fellowship in this sample of clinical researchers was a positive predictor of such funding.

The above studies clearly identify early career research training as a correlate to research activity later in life, although the support for residency-based research training is less common and less well documented than that for fellowship training. In fact, Davis and Kelley (1982) surveyed over 500 M.D. clinical investigators across specialties and found that 66 percent had decided on a research career before completing residency. Additionally, Davis and Kelley found that among 171 respondents who recalled "a particular person or event" as being influential in their career decision, only 11 percent experienced that influence during residency, with 40 percent doing so in medical school and 35 percent after residency. One interpretation of these numbers is that residency is not an important point at which to engage a would-be physician in research training. However, it is equally plausible that the dip reported in residency is the result of the intense clinical demands that occur at that stage, combined with a status quo in residency curriculum that typically involves little research training. From this perspective, residency may represent an untapped opportunity to integrate more research training during a time when career decisions have yet to be completely formed. Accordingly, it appears reasonable to conclude that if fellowship training encourages research career tracking, slightly earlier training might enhance that process, and would be most effective if it simultaneously encouraged residents to pursue research fellowships.

In support of that contention, Neinstein and MacKenzie (1989) found that in a survey of 772 academic physicians, 87 percent had received fellowship research training, and more than 50 percent had received research training during residency and even during medical school. Given the strong linkage found between residency and fellowship research training and the fact that so many who received such training became academicians, early training appears to be an important precursor to a research career. What the study does not conclusively demonstrate is whether these individuals would have gone on to pursue research fellowships in the absence of such early training, nor does it rule out the possibility that fellowship and not residency training is the key factor in predicting an academic career (an issue discussed later in this chapter). Insufficient data exist to judge whether residency-based research training before a fellowship experience makes a significant difference. Nonetheless, it is the strong sense of the committee that the earlier research training occurs the better, and that such training can complement and form a key portion of requisite clinical training because research training (especially in patient-oriented research) is so closely linked to the practice of evidence-based medicine.

Opportunities to Formulate Patient-Oriented Research Questions

Patient-oriented research requires an understanding of the current strengths and weaknesses of clinical care and of emerging technologies that might be used to take that care to a higher level of quality and efficiency. Thus for most psychiatry trainees, residency may be their first opportunity to formulate substantive patient-oriented research questions. Earlier research experiences (e.g., in medical school), especially those that pertain to patient-oriented research, are likely to be less productive for at least two reasons. First, medical students are likely not to have the academic (scientific or clinical) knowledge that residents possess, and thus are less intellectually equipped to formulate contemporary and testable hypotheses. Second, medical students have not served as the primary medical provider to a large number of patients. Such direct patient interactions and responsibilities logically can inspire research questions in the minds of residents, and can also give them a real-world view of the potential impact of advances in patient-oriented research.

Attracting and Sustaining the Interest of Talented Medical Students

Residency training programs that offer research experiences will likely attract medical students with the greatest interest in and ability to pursue research careers. Such students will likely include M.D./Ph.D.'s or equivalently prepared trainees, who traditionally have chosen the more research-intensive specialties, such as internal medicine (Institute of Medicine [IOM], 1994) and neurology (see the discussion of intellectual capacity and scientific orientation in Chapter 5).

Once research-oriented residents have been recruited into psychiatry, it is imperative that they maintain their investigative interests and research skills during the 4- to 5-year residency. The absence of any research experience and lack of exposure to those regularly conducting research during this long period can effectively extinguish any earlier predilection toward such endeavors. This is especially true for M.D./Ph.D. trainees, as research training in a Ph.D. program is typically followed by up to 6 years of clinical training (i.e., medical school and residency) before trainees have the opportunity to reenter research through a fellowship or academic faculty position. Fostering the recruitment and engagement of individuals with an M.D./Ph.D. is important to psychiatric research, as these dual-degree researchers hold 20 to 30 percent of all National Institutes of Health (NIH) grants awarded to physician-scientists, even though they account for less than 2.5 percent of medical school graduates (Association of American Medical Colleges [AAMC], 2002a; Ley and Rosenberg, 2002; Zemlo et al., 2000). Although the committee can cite no empirical data to support the importance of maintaining research skills and interest through inclusion of research experiences in residency, it appears logical that such training would be both practical and encouraging. It furthermore appears that *patient-oriented* research training would serve to keep the trainee abreast of new methodologies and important discoveries entirely germane to competent clinical practice.

IMPORTANCE OF LONGITUDINAL TRAINING FOR POTENTIAL RESEARCHERS

Residency is the committee's focus, but experiences before and after that period are integral and extremely important parts of the entire clinical research training endeavor. Preresidency training (i.e., undergraduate, medical school) and postresidency experiences (i.e., fellowship and junior faculty status) both have a substantial influence on the number of young psychiatrists who choose to engage in patient-oriented research.

While residency clearly constitutes a key crossroads in the career path of many M.D.'s, it represents but one step toward a research career. It is widely acknowledged that more than 2 years of uninterrupted research training is necessary to launch the career of a successful physician-researcher (IOM, 1994; Kimball and Bennett, 1994; Kupfer et al., 2002; Pincus et al., 1995). Given the time that residents must devote to the mastery of clinical skills, research experiences in residency will thus likely provide only a small portion of the overall research training necessary to prepare competent patient-oriented investigators. Accordingly, residency-based research experiences will be most effective if linked to pre- and especially postresidency (i.e., fellowship) training to create an integrated, longitudinal, and thorough research training experience.

Preresidency Experiences

Research experiences during undergraduate education and medical school may shape career preferences. Rancurello (1988) suggests that medical schools that provide a strong psychiatry teaching curriculum, engaging instructors, and training in evidence-based medicine are likely to increase the pool of talented medical students who will be interested in psychiatric research. There are a number of avenues, both formal and informal, through which preresidency trainees can obtain research exposure.

Informal Research Experiences

Undergraduate and, for medical students, preclinical summer research opportunities in psychiatry departments can foster long-term interests among students majoring in related disciplines (e.g., neuroscience, psychology). Medical students may be inspired, alternatively or additionally, to pursue a psychiatric career by the psychiatry clerkship that typically occurs in the third year of medical school (Sierles and Taylor, 1995).

The perception that medical school experiences have an impact on future career choices is strongly supported by the findings of a survey of medical students indicating that approximately 80 percent changed their specialty preference after entering medical school (Kassebaum and Szenas, 1995). An analysis of data from a survey of nearly 500 post–medical school graduates declaring psychiatry as their specialty examined what factors predicted outcomes corresponding to research fellowship and eventual research career plans. Although the magnitude of individual effects is difficult to derive from this analysis, it is apparent that research involvement (as author or investigator) and a research-intensive environment during medical school both were strongly correlated with a new psychiatric resident's desire to pursue a research fellowship and a longer-term research career (Haviland et al., 1987). This study points to the importance of direct and more subtle (e.g., medical school culture) influences on a trainee's career intentions.

Recognizing the importance of recruiting medical students, the disciplines of both internal medicine and neurology have developed student interest groups (i.e., social groups) to educate and attract medical students to their respective specialties (Albritton and Fincher, 1997). Robert Griggs, chair of the Neurology Department, University of Rochester, and editor of *Neurology*, told the committee that such groups not only are inexpensive to run, but also have been important in maintaining a general and a researcher pipeline of neurology students. Several such medical student interest groups also exist in departments of psychiatry, but it is not known how frequently they are used or how successful they are at attracting undergraduates to careers in psychiatric research.

Formal Research Experiences

Formal education programs also exist that support research training in the college or medical school years. The NIH R25 grant mechanism provides funding of up to $150,000 a year over 3 to 5 years for the development of research training curriculum. The University of Pittsburgh (Western Psychiatric Institute and Clinic [WPIC]) and Yale University have both received R25 grants from the National Institute of Mental Health (NIMH). The WPIC program, in collaboration with Carnegie Mellon University, began offering an undergraduate research fellowship in 1994 (Grant No. 5R25MH054318-07). The program selects outstanding junior and senior college students with an interest in postbaccalaureate training in mental health. They are given a small stipend and partial tuition support (WPIC, 2002b). Participants in the year-long program develop a research proposal and conduct supervised clinical or basic research. Trainees also attend two semester-long courses on clinical psychiatry and the neurological bases of psychiatric disorders and participate in a month-long clinical rotation. Participants engage as well in a 14-week-long summer program at WPIC, during which they meet investigators, attend lectures, and visit laboratories. The program enables trainees to obtain in-depth experience in both clinical and basic research in mental health while receiving undergraduate degrees in the neurosciences and the biological, chemical, and psychological sciences. Outcome data from 1994 to 1999 for 65 of 83 trainees indicate that the vast majority (88 percent) received postbaccalaureate training in the health sciences (receiving mainly an M.D. or a Ph.D. in the neurosciences or psychology), and 56 percent published research results within 3 years of completing the program (personal communication, G. Haas, WPIC, April 18, 2003).

The Yale program targets medical students interested in neuroscience research training (Grant No. 5R25MH060477-04). This program, which began in 1999, has a didactic component that again integrates both basic and clinical neuroscience concepts, with case reports, including live patient interviews. Selected students may further take part in a yearlong mentored research experience, which also provides considerable time and support to trainees in developing an individual research project (NIH, 1999a).

Dual-degree programs are increasingly being used to provide medical students and others with formal research training. As of 2002, 37 institutions offered M.D./M.P.H. degrees (AAMC, 2002d). Other programs offer different masters degrees. Wayne State University, for example, offers a master of science in psychiatry to medical students, residents, and fellows; completion of the degree requires supervised research work and a thesis defense (Balon and Kuhn, 2001). Medical students who participate take a year off from their medical schooling. They are funded through a combination of department and senior investigator funds. Since the mid-1990s, three medical students have participated in the program, and all have been first authors of articles and abstracts, made national presentations, and moved on to research-oriented residency training programs; two have attended the American Psychiatric Association's (APA) Research Colloquium (Balon and Kuhn, 2001).

The Medical Scientist Training Program (MSTP) also provides a formal mechanism for research-oriented trainees. Started in 1964, the NIH-funded program provides M.D./Ph.D. trainees with extensive training in laboratory and clinical research over a 7- to 8-year period (AAMC, 1999). M.D./Ph.D. students in the neurosciences are attractive candidates for psychiatry residency and research career tracking (Rancurello, 1988). A web-based review of 13 MSTPs revealed that of 1,133 graduates, 57 (or 5 percent) pursued a residency in psychiatry or received an academic appointment in a psychiatry department.[9] Given that psychiatrists represent approximately 5 percent of all physicians (AAMC, 2002b), it would appear that psychiatry does a reasonable job attracting M.D./Ph.D. students in comparison with other branches of medicine. Nevertheless, increasing the proportion of MSTP graduates entering psychiatry training could have a profound effect on the future of psychiatric research, especially if these new M.D./Ph.D. graduates could be tracked in higher numbers to patient-oriented research careers. Accomplishing this will be challenging, however, since many M.D./Ph.D. trainees pursue basic research careers (AAMC, 1999; Ahrens, 1992; Frieden and Fox, 1991; Sut-

---

[9] Data obtained from the following institutions as of December 20, 2002: University of California, Irvine; University of California, San Diego; Yale University; University of Iowa; University of Michigan; Washington University; Albert Einstein College; Duke University; Case Western Reserve University; Medical University of South Carolina; Baylor College of Medicine; University of Texas Southwestern Medical Center at Dallas; University of Virginia Health System; and Medical College of Wisconsin.

ton and Killian, 1996), while others elect to not continue their research careers after entering the clinical phase of their training.

While the federal government funds a number of initiatives, including the R25 mechanism and the MSTP, foundations also fund preresidency research training. The recently established Doris Duke Clinical Research Fellowship Program offers high-achieving medical students a year of clinical research. Medical students receive a $20,000 stipend, and mentors are given a small stipend for their efforts. The program is administered by 10 selected universities, each of which houses at least 5 fellows. Of the 106 fellows during 2001 and 2002, 15 were involved in neuroscience and 6 in psychiatry. Appendix B lists other funding opportunities for individuals and programs interested in developing their research training portfolios (the appendix is organized by career stage and is designed to be illustrative rather than exhaustive).

Postresidency Experiences

Residency is very rigorous, leaving limited opportunity to engage in patient-oriented research. This is particularly true for residents who receive clinical subspecialty fellowship training. Research training is usually not integrated with child and adolescent psychiatry training or with postresidency fellowship training in geriatric, addiction, forensic, and consultation-liaison psychiatry (Pincus et al., 1995). Training in child and adolescent psychiatry, for instance, typically requires a 5-year residency (3 years of adult [general] psychiatry and 2 years of subspecialty training in child and adolescent psychiatry) and is clinically intensive, and most programs allocate only about 4 months for elective activities (see the discussion of the Psychiatry Residency Review Committee in Chapter 3).

While some new psychiatrists can move directly from residency to academic positions, most who wish to become independent researchers enroll in additional training. Indeed, further preparation for research careers (in the form of a fellowship) is usually essential for individuals who wish to conduct independent psychiatric research. As noted earlier in this chapter, Pincus et al. (1995) found a significant, positive correlation between fellowship training and psychiatric research career involvement among M.D.'s. They also found a "dose-response" association of sorts, as the length of that training was positively correlated with subsequent research involvement for all single-degree doctorate holders (i.e., M.D. or Ph.D. alone, but not M.D./Ph.D.). Using a survey of 117 (78 percent response rate) early- to mid-career pediatricians with a track record of one publication per year for the 5-year sample period from 1976 to 1981, Ledley and Lovejoy (1993) found that, aside from Ph.D.-training and an interest in research, fellowship or other postdoctoral training was a dominant factor in encouraging young pediatricians to pursue research and in providing those trainees with the skills necessary to be successful in doing so. More than 75 percent of the respondents indicated that this training beyond residency "strongly stimulated" their ability to do research. By comparison, fewer than 50 percent of the sample cited their residency training or technical or scientific background as having the same positive impact. These data can be taken to indicate that postresidency fellowship training is an important segue for many new physicians entering research—one that the trainees themselves recognize as central. Central to the theme of this report is the need to recruit more psychiatrists into research fellowships. It is likely that research exposure in residency can be one way to enhance that recruitment effort.

Masters Programs

Masters programs are available for postdoctoral fellows at a number of institutions. The Mayo Clinic, for example, offers residents and fellows a masters degree in biomedical science or clinical research through the Clinician-Investigator Training Program, which includes a journal club, tutorials, and seminars and supports 2 years of uninterrupted research time (Mayo Graduate School of Medicine, 2002). Recent data from that program indicate that 75 percent of graduates receive at least some extramural funding for their research, but that number drops to 50 percent if one considers how many of these graduates are able to fund more than half of their research activities with extramural funds. As of April 2003, there were 93 program graduates, but none were psychiatrists (personal communication, M. Rieder, Mayo Graduate School of Medicine, April 10, 2003).

Emory University offers a master of science as part of its Clinical Research Curriculum Award Program (a K12 federally funded program) for fellows and junior faculty. The 2-year program offers courses in statistics, research design, epidemiology, scientific writing, and bioethics. It further requires the completion of a mentored thesis and aims to equip trainees to prepare an application for an NIH career award (Emory School of Medicine, 2000). As of April 2003, only a total of 3 psychiatrists have enrolled in this K12 program. The other two are expected to graduate by 2006 (personal communication, C. Sroka, Emory University, June 23, 2003).

T32 Funding Mechanism

Another mechanism for supporting postdoctoral training of psychiatrists is the federal T32 grant mechanism. Columbia University has T32 grants in several areas, including schizophrenia and affective disorders, to train psychiatry residents. A key goal of these programs is to provide fellows the time and training to apply for an early mentored career or K award (see below). The didactic curriculum includes research design, ethics, modern research techniques, and statistics. The fellowship lasts 2 to 3 years, and stipends are subsidized in part by state funds (Rieder, 2001). Of 42 fellows who completed training in either schizophrenia or affective disorders from 1989 to 1998, 19 (or 45 percent) have received K awards, and another 10 conduct full-time psychiatric research (Rieder, 2003). Of these 29 individuals, the vast majority (86 percent) are said to be conducting clinical or clinical neuroscience research (Rieder, 2003).

The University of Colorado has a T32 grant to increase the number of academic child and adolescent psychiatrist researchers. The 2-year postdoctoral program, which has been in existence since 1980 and currently operates under the auspices of the Developmental Psychobiology Research Group of the department of psychiatry, is available to M.D.'s and Ph.D.'s. Trainees receive formal instruction, participate in seminars, attend retreats, and are expected to complete an independent research project and submit a career development award (University of Colorado, 2002). Since 1978, 98 postdoctoral trainees have enrolled in the program, 26 of whom were psychiatrists. Of the 9 child and adolescent psychiatrists who have completed the program, 8 are active researchers and academics (personal communication, L. Greco-Sanders, University of Colorado, August 7, 2003).

As a complement to T32 or other training grants (e.g., fellowship grants), programs should consider the NIH K30 mechanism, which provides resources for the development of a curriculum designed to train individuals across medical and nonmedical disciplines in the methods of clinical research (see Chapter 4 and Appendix B). In a way, the K30 can be viewed as infrastructure support for clinical research training, while T32 and other such grants support individual matriculants. Individuals who wish to pursue extended postdoctoral fellowship training may consider the NIH-funded fellowship (F32) that provides a stipend of at least $34,000 for extended training in biomedical and behavioral research (see Appendix B for further information). Unfortunately, the data suggest that the number of M.D.'s receiving an F32 fellowship declined by 43 percent from 1985 to 1997 (Zemlo et al., 2000).

Private Funding Mechanisms

Private foundations and professional societies offer a number of research fellowships in psychiatric research. Two exemplary research training fellowships for psychiatrists are the National Alliance for Research on Schizophrenia and Depression's (NARSAD) Young Investigator Award and The Robert Wood Johnson Foundation's Clinical Scholars Program. NARSAD's award provides up to $30,000 for 1 to 2 years for fellows and junior faculty to conduct research pertaining to major mental disorders, including schizophrenia and affective disorders. NARSAD funded 175 junior investigator awards in 2003 (NARSAD, 2002; 2003).

The program of The Robert Wood Johnson Foundation is aimed at young physicians who are committed to medicine and are interested in the acquisition of new skills and training in the nonbiological sciences important to medical care systems, including epidemiology and health services research. The 2-year fellowship is supported by a stipend of about $44,000 and requires the completion of graduate-level work, with up to 20 percent of a fellow's time being devoted to maintaining clinical skills. Fellows in the program reside at one of seven universities, each with its own priority area (e.g., evaluating health care practices and interventions at The Johns Hopkins University, or improving the care of America's at-risk populations at the University of California, Los Angeles). Former scholars are involved in academic (60 percent) and clinical (13 percent) medicine or public policy. As of July 2002, nearly 900 scholars, including more than 80 psychiatrists, had completed the program (The Robert Wood Johnson Foundation, 2001).

A small number of fellowships supported by the pharmaceutical industry are coordinated by professional societies, such as the APA's American Psychiatric Institute of Research and Education (APIRE) and the American College of Neuropsychopharmacology. Additionally, since 1989 the APA has administered the T32-supported Program for Minority Research Training in Psychiatry, which funds research experiences from medical school through postresidency fellowships (see the discussion of underrepresented racial and ethnic minorities in Chapter 5). Residents may pursue various areas of investigation, including schizophrenia, neuroscience, and child psychiatry (APA, 2002d). As of 2002, 45 of the 58 graduates of this T32 program held an academic or research position, had received 109 grants/awards, and had authored more than 400 journal articles and books. Of the remaining 13 graduates, who are affiliated primarily with a private practice, many have published articles or received grants (personal communication, E. Guerra, APA, December 4, 2002).

APIRE also collaborates with pharmaceutical companies. For instance, APIRE and Eli Lilly sponsor a 1-year fellowship for trainees who have completed their psychiatric residency. Initiated in 1988, the award provides a $45,000 stipend, and fellows are required to spend 85 percent of their time doing research (APA, 2002a). APIRE also collaborates with Wyeth Pharmaceuticals, Janssen Pharmaceuticals, and GlaxoSmithKline to fund similar fellowships. In fact, of the 12 APA awards listed on the APIRE website, all but 2 are funded in part by pharmaceutical companies (see Appendix B for further description of funding opportunities available through professional societies).

Despite the availability and successes of research fellowship programs, such programs often are not utilized (Kimball, 1994; Whitcomb and Walter, 2000; Zemlo et al., 2000). For instance, Whitcomb and Walter (2000) found that only 2 percent of subspecialty fellows entered the research-oriented American Board of Internal Medicine (ABIM) pathway (discussed further below), despite efforts to enroll as many as 10 percent of such fellows. Likewise, Zemlo et al. (2000) found that physicians do not track to additional fellowship training, in part because of lengthened training in preparation for a research career and limited stipends. Low financial compensation no doubt offers some explanation for why residents do not pursue fellowships in increasing numbers. Fellowships add time to training, and they do so while offering salaries below what clinicians with the same experience earn. Specifically, the average fellowship stipend is $40,000 to $50,000, whereas clinical salaries are double or triple that amount.[10] Given this financial disincentive to engage in research training, it is especially important that fellowship experiences be linked practically and conceptually to residency. Practical linkage means appropriate financial aid to those who qualify; conceptual linkage means demonstrating to the resident that there is light at the end of the tunnel in the form of junior and senior research career awards (see below) that can offset the short-term sacrifices in salary (see Chapter 5 for a discussion of personal finances).

Early Mentored Career Awards

Beyond fellowship, or even in the late stages of fellowship, potential psychiatrist-investigators can benefit greatly from early mentored career

---

[10]The average entry-level salary for a psychiatrist in New York State was $120,000 in 2001 (Nolan et al., 2002); nationally, the mean salary for psychiatrists in 2001 was $114,000 (Bureau of Labor Statistics, 2002).

awards (K awards). This NIH funding mechanism provides salary support to a maximum of $90,000 per year for up to 5 years. Under the supervision of a designated mentor, awardees are expected to commit 75 percent of their time to a research project, and they are provided protected time to acquire skills and conduct their own research, which leads them to achieve the status of independent investigator. One of the long-term goals of K awardees is to progress to principal investigator status on research grants such as NIH R01's.

NIMH recently reviewed the achievements of 241 K awardees who received funding between 1989 and 2000, including active (n = 163) and completed (n = 78) grants (personal communication, A. Permell and W. Goldschmidts, NIMH, December 12, 2002). Of these awardees, 119 had applied for an R01 grant, and 62 (52 percent) had been funded. A separate review of 31 early research career awardees (K awards and the discontinued R29 or "FIRST" award) in geriatric/aging mental health research was recently conducted using the public Computer Retrieval of Information on Scientific Projects (CRISP) database (Bruce, 2002). More than 40 percent of individuals who had completed their early career awards between 1997 and 2001 had obtained R01 grants. Given that success rates for psychiatrists on K awards in recent years have been at least 40 percent—similar to those for other mental health professionals, such as psychologists[11]—an ambitious psychiatrist can consider the path from K award to R01 an attainable career goal.

At the same time, it is reasonable to ask why as many as 60 percent of K awardees do not appear to move to the next level of the federal grant pipeline. Some certainly carry on their research as coinvestigators or as investigators on foundation- or industry-sponsored projects, so that the 60 percent "failure" rate for K awardees is likely overestimated. Others, however, simply do not go on to become productive researchers. Given that a 5-year K award involves a federal investment that can easily exceed $500,000 per awardee, it is imperative that studies be done to understand why the failure rate in mentored research training is so high. One potentially useful way to conduct such studies would be to survey the trainees and mentors who fail at the intended transition of K award to R01, and compare their experiences and attributes with those of the individuals who succeed.

---

[11]Raw data courtesy of the NIMH, Office of Science Policy and Program Policy, February 21, 2003. Analysis done by IOM staff.

IOM outreach to K awardees. To understand some of the concerns of today's K awardees, the committee interviewed seven randomly selected[12] psychiatrist-investigators who had received K awards since 1998 (see Appendix B). Not surprisingly, interviewees noted that limited time and money were their two chief concerns. One respondent complained that research time is often taken up by administrative and clinical responsibilities, leaving little time to read, think, and write. Nearly all respondents noted limited protected time for research, low salaries relative to those of full-time clinicians, and general uncertainty about continued funding. Good mentoring, hard work, a supportive spouse/partner and/or department chair, and a strong interest in research and writing were factors commonly cited as helping to overcome the obstacles to a research career. Unfortunately, the confidentiality requirements of NIMH prevented the committee from making parallel inquiries of individuals whose K applications had not been approved and who had chosen not to resubmit or further pursue a career development award. Consequently, it is not clear what factors, personal or professional, prevented them from obtaining federal funding.

AAMC and NIH outreach to K23 awardees. The K23 is a relatively new NIH award, designed specifically to offer mentored training for patient-oriented researchers. For strategic planning purposes, AAMC and NIH hired a market research firm to conduct three focus groups with approximately 30 awardees in March 2001. The results obtained from those focus groups were very similar to those of the outreach described above. The K23 recipients were concerned principally about time and money. Time limitations were imposed largely by clinical demands, although some frustration with regulations related to clinical research (e.g., protection of human subjects) was also noted. Academic institutions were characterized as interested in research, but not forthcoming with support in the form of resources and true protected time for funded or intramural research efforts. Although protected time was a central theme among these respondents, it is interesting that they did not suggest that their departments or institutions needed to be more respectful of their 75 percent protected time (a requirement of the K23 award). Instead, they recommended that a K23 award be available that would cover 50 percent research time so awardees could spend the remaining 50 percent on clinical work. Although most respondents were enthusiastic about submitting

---

[12]K award recipients in psychiatry were identified using the federal CRISP database (NIH, 1999a) and randomly selected from that list.

future applications for federal grants, especially R01 grants, most also expressed the need for additional bridge funding between the K23 and a large independent research grant. Details of this bridge and the reason it would be necessary after 5 years of training support, however, were not explored (Henderson et al., 2001). Despite these limitations, the K23 was noted as a good jump-start for a clinical research career. Focus groups were not conducted with individuals whose K awards had not been funded and who had chosen not to pursue further resubmission.

STRATEGIC CONSIDERATIONS

Early planning can allow for useful connectivity between residency and fellowship, and then to career awards. In particular, those interested in research-intensive careers should consider research fellowship training as early as possible during residency, since, as noted previously, early research experiences are known to be correlated with research career tracking (Davis and Kelley, 1982; Dial et al., 1990; Dunn et al., 1998; Haviland et al., 1987; Pincus et al., 1993; Ringel et al., 2001). Opportunities for residents to participate in research and to continue such endeavors into fellowship in the same department have the advantage of providing a more cohesive longitudinal research training period—one that is often preferable to two or more fragmented research training periods. The utility of this approach is supported by the reality that the best residents are encouraged to remain as fellows in the departments in which they have trained.

Given the clinical responsibilities and goals of residency, most programs offer few if any direct research experiences to the large majority of residents (see the discussion of program and curriculum structure in Chapter 4). Accordingly, research fellowship training is often the first concentrated and practical research experience encountered by a psychiatrist. It is also one that can provide a realistic transition to junior faculty status.

This multistep career path will likely not be obvious to trainees themselves, who are preoccupied with the academic, clinical, and core paperwork demands that must be met to transition from one training phase to the next. Therefore, some programs have developed and promoted a departmental culture aimed at funding research training at all career stages. For example, WPIC has created a portfolio of grants and discretionary funds to ensure that research training is supported at all educational stages, including the requirement that a large number of faculty have senior career or independent research awards (Pincus, 2002;

Pincus et al., 1993) (see Table 2-1). Given WPIC's success (it receives the highest level of NIH funding among psychiatry departments[13]), the development of similar multilayered grant portfolios should be attempted by other programs. Even if such a multistage strategy can be implemented only on a small scale (e.g., one or two funded slots at each career stage), it has the potential to familiarize both institutions and trainees with the fullest range of funding options across the research workforce pipeline.

Models from Outside of Psychiatry

Although pediatrics and internal medicine have far from solved their own problems of attracting residents to research careers, these two disciplines have created pathways that link residency training with 2- or 3-year research-intensive fellowships. The connection is made by offering

TABLE 2-1 Western Psychiatric Institute and Clinic's Developmental Pathway for Psychiatric Researchers

Duration of Training (years)	Stage of Education	Funding Mechanism[a]
4	Undergraduate	R25 research grant
4	Medical school	T32 training grant, Medical Scientist Training Program
4	Residency	Research track (department funded)
2	Fellowship	T32 training grant
2	Junior faculty (1)	R25 research grant
5	Junior faculty (2)	Career (K) award
--	Senior faculty	Career (K) award, Research (R) grant, Project (P) grant

NOTE: [a] National Institutes of Health unless otherwise noted.
SOURCE: Pincus (2002)

---

[13] Nearly $78 million in fiscal year 2002.

residents the opportunity to shorten their general residency training by 12 months if they commit to extra research and subspecialty training of 2 to 4 years. The ABIM research pathway, known as the Clinical Investigator Pathway (CIP), requires that enrolled fellows spend 80 percent of their time engaged in research training, leaving the other 20 percent for clinical service (ABIM, 2002). A review of two institutions that offered a CIP—Brigham Young University and Massachusetts General Hospital—indicates that more than 75 percent of program graduates remained in research careers (Kimball, 1994). A more recent review, however, notes two significant problems with the program. First, despite the mandate for 80 percent research time, fellows, even at academic centers, typically are able to devote only 50 percent of their time to research because of their institution's clinical demands. Second, and more disturbing, it appears that this program is recruiting trainees at rates far below those projected—2 percent rather than 10 percent of all subspecialty fellows (Whitcomb and Walter, 2000). These realities suggest that the incentives associated with the pathway are not keeping pace with clinical revenue and other pressures steering trainees away from research careers.

For pediatrics, research training has been combined with subspecialty training (i.e., not available to general pediatrics residents) (American Board of Pediatrics [ABP], 2001; 2002a; 2002b). Additionally, ABP recently approved several pathways—including the Integrated Research Pathway and the Subspecialty Fast Track Pathway—that allow early integration of research into residency for those with previous research experience (e.g., M.D./Ph.D. degree holders), as well as the Special Alternative Pathway, for those who achieve clinical competency at an accelerated pace. Most of these pathways offer some time incentive to trainees such that if they commit to research training, they can complete some of the core training requirements in less time or engage in research training earlier than standard pathway residents.

Table 2-2 summarizes these pathways, along with the previously established Pediatric Scientist Development Program (PSDP). All, with the exception of the PSDP, are too new for any outcome information to be available. The PSDP is a 6- to 7-year pathway that adds 3 to 4 years of research fellowship onto standard residency training. It also offers trainees the possibility of assuming a junior faculty position once they graduate. A 2002 review of 89 PSDP fellows found that 94 percent were faculty in academic pediatric departments, and many of those graduates had also obtained federal research grants. Specifically, 42 PSDP graduates who entered the program from 1987 to 1991 had obtained 35 federal grants, including 21 R01 grants, as of 2001 (Hostetter, 2002). Further evidence indicates that PSDP trainees who receive 3 years of fellowship support may be more likely to receive NIH grants than those trainees who receive 2 years of fellowship funding. Specifically, between 1987 and 2001, 23 of 64 individuals with third-year fellowship funding received federal grant monies, compared with 5 individuals with 2 years of funding. The partial success of this program has encouraged pediatrics to develop the new, accelerated pathways described above. It is hoped that the new programs will attract and retain more researchers by tailoring the training duration to the research and clinical aptitude of the enrollees.

TABLE 2-2 Duration in Years of the Two Stages of Pediatric Subspecialty Training Pathways Outlined by the American Board of Pediatrics and the Pediatric Scientist Development Program

| Activity | Standard Pathway (years) | Pathways for Those with Significant Prior Research Experience (years) | | Special Alternative Pathway (years) | Pediatric Scientist Development Program (years) |
		Integrated Research Pathway[a]	Subspecialty Fast Track Pathway[b]		
General Pediatrics Residency	3	3 (1 year for research)	3	2[c]	2-3[d]
Subspecialty and Research Training	3	3	2	3	3-4[e]
Total Time	6	6	5	5	5-7[f]

NOTES:
[a] For M.D./Ph.D. graduates or students with significant research experience.
[b] For students with considerable research experience, e.g., Ph.D. or publication record.
[c] Residents must pass an examination at the end of the first year of general pediatric training to permit reduction of general training from 3 to 2 years.
[d] Residents who complete training in 2 years must declare themselves "fast trackers" and are required to pass an examination at the end of the first year of general pediatric training to permit reduction of training to 2 years.
[e] Training includes 1 year of clinical training and 2-3 years of exclusive research training.
[f] Fellows are given assistance in identifying a junior faculty position that will provide 2 years of support with 75 percent time for research.
SOURCE: American Board of Pediatrics (2002a); Hostetter (2002)

Both the internal medicine and pediatrics programs described above operate on the principle that general training can be shortened as an incentive to qualified individuals committed to further subspecialty clinical training and extended research training. Shortening of general training is based on two premises. First, superior trainees master clinical skills quickly enough to obviate the need for longer core training. Second, trainees will make up for lost clinical exposure during their subspecialty training (i.e., patient interactions in the context of clinical research and subspecialty clinical service). Additionally, it should be noted that clinical time in fellowship will likely be maximized for patient-oriented researchers, although the programs described are available to those engaged in basic research as well.

CONCLUSIONS AND RECOMMENDATION 2.1

Residency is a pivotal interval in psychiatric training. It represents an opportunity to educate all residents for the lifelong practice of evidence-based medicine, to provide some residents with initial research experiences that may launch them on a career of patient-oriented research, and to sustain the research interests of trainees with previous research experience (e.g., M.D./Ph.D.'s). Programs that link residency research training to preceding and subsequent experiences by establishing programmatic and funding pathways will likely ensure the best research training outcomes. Research training programs developed by ABIM and ABP are models for the more direct connection of residency to fellowship research training experiences. To facilitate connectivity between residency and research fellowship in psychiatry, the committee makes the following recommendation:

> **Recommendation 2.1. Departments of psychiatry should organize optional research experiences and mandatory research didactics in residency as early steps in research career development pathways, leading from residency to a junior faculty appointment. Federal and private agencies should expand mechanisms that encourage psychiatry trainees to enter and move, without interruption, from residency to a research fellowship to a faculty position, all designed to promote independence as a patient-oriented investigator.**

This recommendation targets the residency-to-fellowship portion of the training path because fellowship training has the best track record and because post–medical school training experiences are immediately proximal to the point at which a physician matures to vocational independence. At the same time, it should be noted that these fellowships often have not succeeded in attracting the numbers of trainees needed to sustain the physician-researcher workforce. Consequently, early experiences (e.g., medical school–based research exposure) described in this chapter will likely be important in attracting more psychiatrists to patient-oriented research careers. In residency, research tracks (see Chapter 4) are clearly one way to offer special experiences to individuals who commit early to research training paths during residency. In addition, mandatory research didactic learning (e.g., lectures and reading of epidemiology, study design, clinical consent procedures, grant preparation) for all residents may well have the dual benefit of enhancing evidence-based practice and promoting research interest among some residents who might otherwise not consider research careers.

3

Regulatory Factors

The previous chapter addressed research training and research exposures that occur before and after residency. This and the next two chapters focus more directly on the residency experience. This chapter details how residency programs, and residents themselves, are regulated by national governing bodies that are designed to ensure that all training programs meet minimal standards, and that all individual trainees attain the necessary skills and knowledge to be certified as psychiatrists. The chapter describes several national professional societies that, in one form or another, have an interest in residency-based training. The impact of these organizations on research training outcomes in residency is addressed. The chapter ends with conclusions and recommendations.

PSYCHIATRY RESIDENCY REVIEW COMMITTEE

Organization and Function

The Psychiatry Residency Review Committee (RRC) is the organization with principal responsibility for setting the minimal standards and content for adult and child and adolescent psychiatry residency training programs. It, along with 24 other medical specialty RRCs, operates under the aegis of the nonprofit and volunteer-driven Accreditation Council for Graduate Medical Education (ACGME, 2002a). As of 2003, the Psychiatry RRC had 18 members. The committee's members are appointed by or sit as ex officio members from one of the following three organizations: the American Board of Psychiatry and Neurology (ABPN), the Council of Medical Education of the American Medical Association (AMA), and the American Psychiatric Association (APA). The ACGME requires that members of an RRC "have demonstrated substantial experience in administrative and/or teaching within the specialty" to qualify for service. Each RRC also includes a single member who is a resident in the appropriate specialty. Appointments are made for 3 years, and members' terms are limited to 6 years. No provisions exist that specifically require the membership of researchers on the RRC (ACGME, 2002c), and at least two recent Psychiatry RRC chairs have said that researchers do not tend to be members and are not typically involved in the committee's periodic revision of the written requirements for residency program accreditation (Miller, 2002; Winstead, 2002).

The principal responsibility of the psychiatry RRC is to review and accredit individual programs by checking documentation and making site visits to ensure compliance with the requirements set by the committee. Programs found in violation may be cited, and in extreme cases, their accreditation may be suspended or revoked. The accreditation process is designed to safeguard the public by maintaining necessary clinical standards in psychiatric graduate medical education. Additionally, the RRC must evaluate and update the written requirements for residency programs at least every 5 years. The requirements contain a lengthy description of the environment, curriculum, and overall procedures to which departments of psychiatry must conform to be accredited as a residency program in the United States.

Accreditation has a direct bearing on two important aspects of graduate medical education. First, one must graduate from an accredited program to qualify for professional board certification as an adult (general) or child and adolescent psychiatrist or in any of the other recognized subspecialties (such as geriatric psychiatry, forensic psychiatry, addiction psychiatry, and pain management). Second, program accreditation is necessary if training institutions are to qualify for federal funding that supports resident stipends, as well as other costs associated with graduate medical education (see the discussion of graduate medical education funding in Chapter 4).

In formulating program requirements, the Psychiatry RRC aims to represent the entire field of U.S. psychiatry as broadly and equitably as possible, with regard to both different branches of practice (e.g., geriatrics, addiction, forensics) and different sizes of programs (Miller, 2002). Although this universal approach permits a thorough formulation of training requirements, it also has a tendency to result in requirements that continually expand, thereby encroaching upon elective time during which a resident might choose to engage in hands-on or more intensive research training. This tendency to add onto existing mandates also appears to have been at least partially responsible for the controversial introduction of a psychodynamic psychotherapy requirement in the recent revision of the RRC requirements that took effect in early 2001.

A public exchange between then RRC chair (Daniel Winstead) and then head of the National Institute of Mental Health (NIMH) (Steven Hyman) demonstrates the tension that has arisen because of these requirements, and furthermore highlights the fact that the RRC process is at least in part a political one. The exchange took place during Dr. Winstead's presentation on training requirements to a small group of experts convened by NIMH and the APA to discuss the general problem of research training in the field of psychiatry (Winstead, 2001). Below is an extract from transcripts of that meeting, which occurred in November 2001. At the time, Dr. Winstead was describing the five psychotherapy requirements mandated by the RRC for all psychiatric training programs as of January 2001. One of the five is psychodynamic psychotherapy.

> *Dr. Hyman:* Dan, I'm sorry to interrupt. I just want to highlight this for later discussion. Of course, we support a lot of psychotherapy research, and we would all agree that psychotherapy is absolutely critical. I mean, if you had a heart attack and somebody just wrote you a script [sic] and didn't prescribe psychosocial rehabilitative exercise and interventions, that would be bad medicine. So the problems with psychotherapy are very complicated. It's interesting that you have psychodynamic therapy up there, and I flag that as a problem. In my five-and-a-half years as NIMH director, we've not had a single application come in to study psychodynamic therapy. So in essence, whatever we think historically, you have as a requirement something for which there is no acceptable evidence, and I think we have to, as a field, grapple with what it means that you have succumbed to historical and collegial pressures and have put up as a requirement something that is not evidence-based and for which the practitioners are not even, by NIMH application standards, interested in being in the game. I just want to highlight that because I think it's a very important point.

> *Dr. Winstead:* It is an important point, and I might tell you that as part of the process, at one point the program requirements went out where we said that the program should pick...[three of][14] these five. I wanted to say that. That's when we heard in spades from the psychodynamic psychotherapy community about the...
>
> *Dr. Hyman:* Sure. They're protecting their livelihood....But the issue is, are we sending a message that...we're going to require something for which there is no evidence?

This exchange clearly demonstrates the reality that preferences rooted in traditional psychiatric practice play a role in both the conception and revision of residency training requirements. The psychiatric research community also must be prepared to engage in the residency training debate, at least to the extent that it is relevant to optimal residency-based research training and the steady evolution of psychiatry as an evidence-based medical discipline. As controversy appears inevitable, the next section detours briefly into a discussion of psychodynamics and considers how it is relevant to residency training and research training. This detour is considered important because the committee is aware of many in the field of psychiatry who are concerned about the inclusion and others about the exclusion of psychodynamic psychotherapy on the competency list for trainees. How this tension is managed has implications for the quantity and quality of research opportunities in psychiatric residency.

A Brief Detour into Psychodynamic Psychotherapy

Psychodynamic psychotherapy encompasses specific forms of psychotherapy (e.g., talk therapy) involving the application of a variety of theories regarding the psychological adaptive processes that have evolved throughout an individual's development and that occur at varying levels of conscious awareness. These theories are based largely on conceptions of how early and later adverse life events impact emotions, memories, personality development, and characteristic coping strategies. They often focus on psychological attitudes that conflict with one an-

---

[14] Correction verified per personal communication, D. Winstead, Chair, Department of Psychiatry and Neurology, Tulane University, April 7, 2003.

other. Treatments may be long-term (years), and even shorter-term psychodynamic-based psychotherapies may extend for many months.

Although the evidence base for these psychotherapies is weak, new studies and meta-analyses of existing data suggest that some of them may be effective for a variety of psychiatric disorders, including personality disorders (Leichsenring and Leibing, 2003). However, as expressed by Dr. Hyman in the dialogue at the close of the previous section of this report, as well as by other prominent psychiatrists (Eisenberg, 2002; Kandel, 1998), there is concern in the field of psychiatry that the traditional psychotherapies associated with psychodynamics are not sufficiently evidence-based, making their inclusion on the competency list for psychiatry training questionable. Accordingly, some argue that psychodynamic competency training represents a poor use of training resources (especially time), and that it further may drive scientifically oriented trainees away from the practice of psychiatry (see the discussion of intellectual capacity and scientific orientation in Chapter 5). This concern about recruiting scientifically oriented students likely stems from the fact that psychodynamic theory is strongly linked to case studies developed over a century ago (by Sigmund Freud), and based on clinical experience (rather than systematic study) since that time.

Conversely, advocates of psychodynamic approaches argue that such methods represent a valuable aspect of psychiatry that not only is part of the field's uniquely humanistic and patient-centered approach, but also offers a necessary balance to current over-reliance on "quick-fix" remedies (e.g., psychopharmacologic treatment, short-term psychotherapy) for problems that may have complex behavioral and sociologic antecedents (Braslow, 2002). Even well-respected neuroscientists acknowledge that psychodynamics is among "...the most coherent and intellectually satisfying view[s] of the mind" (Kandel, 1999:505), while others, including critics, praise psychodynamics for helping "...psychiatry preserve an abiding interest in the individuality of patients..." (Eisenberg, 2002:32). And most importantly, contemporary research clearly reveals how genetic vulnerabilities interact with life events to yield such devastating mental illnesses as depression (Caspi et al., 2003), suggesting that therapies focused on helping patients understand and better cope with negative experiences are likely to be valuable in treating these disorders.

For this report, the committee felt compelled by numerous suggestions from outside its ranks to consider whether the inclusion of psychodynamics as an explicit residency training requirement represents an impediment to psychiatric research training. Despite some concern that the psychodynamic requirement does emphasize a commitment to a method with a limited evidence base, the committee ultimately decided that the concern about psychodynamics is more a "red herring" with regard to research training in psychiatry than a major issue of concern. The committee is concerned only marginally about the inclusion of a psychodynamic competency requirement for two reasons. First, the committee believes that psychiatrists today are keenly aware of the complexities of treating mental disorders using both psychosocial and psychopharmacologic strategies. Second, the committee is optimistic that impartial research will continue to differentiate therapies according to their effectiveness, but that sound clinical judgment may still be required to provide pragmatic guidance for psychiatric education and practice.

The committee's strong professional impression is that the vast majority of today's psychiatrists realize that there are both effective biological (e.g., drugs) and psychological therapies for many major mental disorders (see Chapter 1 for a review), and that competent practice requires appropriate selection and use of each or both depending on the clinical situation. It is for this reason that Dr. Hyman noted in the above excerpt that sole reliance on a pharmacologic prescription, even for cardiovascular disease, would be "bad medicine." Although the committee's impression is not based on systematic surveys of active psychiatrists, detailed historical review of psychiatric practice demonstrates that psychiatry has emerged as an integrated brain and behavioral discipline since the middle of the twentieth century, when psychodynamics dominated the field (Braslow, 2002). Similarly, and related to the progression of psychiatry, is the evolution of the nature/nurture debate in the behavioral sciences. Regarding that more far-reaching debate, the committee believes that great progress has occurred such that disagreements between those espousing biological determinism and those arguing for the supreme importance of upbringing and social environment have in many ways been transformed into a collaboration—that collaboration being based on a large body of research in recent years that has eloquently demonstrated the influence of both innate genetics and external factors, including psychosocial ones, on behavioral and emotional health (Pinker, 2003).

In considering the potential resistance that might ensue from criticism of psychodynamic psychotherapies, one should not confuse psychodynamic psychotherapies with all forms of psychotherapy, and one should also realize that a number of different forms of psychotherapy that deal with conflicts, defense mechanisms, and maladaptive reactions to adverse life events fall under the general rubric of psychodynamic psychotherapy. There are at least seven other schools of psychotherapy that have been codified (Beitman and Yue, 1999). Even if psychodynamics were eliminated altogether from psychiatric training—something the committee considers neither reasonable nor probable—other psychotherapeutic approaches would remain important aspects of psychiatric knowledge and practice. This point is made explicitly because the practice of psychiatry in recent years has shifted as a result of the impact of neuropharmacologic advances, as well as cost-saving strategies in mental health that often involve psychotherapy delivery by lower-paid professionals (i.e., psychologists and masters-level therapists rather than psychiatrists) (Olfson et al., 1999). A suggestion that psychodynamic psychotherapies be deemphasized in residency training is not, at least in the committee's view, linked to shifting psychiatry from a brain and behavioral discipline to one more focused on neuroscience. Instead, such a suggestion is intended to encourage psychiatry as a field to emphasize to residents evidence-based therapeutic strategies that broadly, but objectively, span both the biological and psychosocial interventions that compose psychiatric practice and make it a viable discipline.

Finally, with regard to psychodynamic psychotherapies, psychiatric educators should keep in mind that psychiatry is not alone in the broad use of techniques that have not been empirically validated (Eisenberg, 2002). Some estimate that 85 percent of all medical therapies are widely used without having undergone some form of systematic, nonbiased testing (Millenson, 1998). This is likely the case because clinical trials are not easily accomplished, and in some cases may be unnecessary in the face of overwhelming evidence obtained in less systematic ways. This high percentage of unvalidated techniques, however, also points to the need for increasing patient-oriented research and research training toward the ultimate goal of optimizing the practice of evidence-based medicine (Institute of Medicine [IOM], 2001a). Psychiatry, like all branches of medicine, needs to remain vigilant against traditional therapies that not only waste resources, but also can harm rather than heal patients. Such medical fallibility appears to have been exposed recently by a randomized, blind trial of arthroscopic surgery for degenerative arthritis in the knee—a procedure that is performed on 650,000 individuals each year (Moseley et al., 2002). In the absence of complete knowledge, professional disciplines such as psychiatry can decide that certain types of practice are worthy of continued practice and corresponding resident training, and for the moment, psychodynamic psychotherapy may be one of those practices. Alternatively, however, such therapy, along with other theories and practices with a limited evidence base, might be deemphasized to accommodate other educational priorities, including research training.

The deemphasis of psychodynamic methods should furthermore be coupled with psychodynamic research and research training by those skilled or interested in such methods. Better evaluation of psychodynamic techniques has been advocated by members of the psychodynamic community (Gabbard et al., 2002). More generally with regard to psychiatric practice, comprehensive increases in *evidence-based* mental health care have been strongly recommended by a high-profile federal commission (New Freedom Commission on Mental Health, 2003).

Clinical Requirements for Psychiatry Training

To understand some of the details regarding the Psychiatry RRC and research training, the committee spoke directly with the last two RRC chairs—Sheldon I. Miller, M.D., and Daniel K. Winstead, M.D.—and carefully reviewed and compared the Psychiatry RRC guidelines with those of selected other medical specialties. The committee also spoke with Stephen I. Wasserman, past chair of the American Board of Allergy and Immunology (A&I), to gain insight into the regulatory process that pertains to A&I and internal medicine, as the latter is the foundation of the former.

As context for discussion of the Psychiatry RRC requirements, the time and research requirements of clinical training for several specialties and subspecialties are summarized in Table 3-1. Residency training for adult (general) psychiatry is 4 years, 1 year longer than that for general internal medicine and on par with that for several other specialties, including neurology and pathology. Residency training for child and adolescent psychiatry is 5 years (typically composed of 3 years of adult [general] training followed by 2 years of child and adolescent training), placing it on par with A&I training. The committee selected A&I for comparison because a high proportion (9.8 percent) of its subspecialists claim research as a primary activity (Association of American Medical Colleges [AAMC], 2002b). Pulmonology/critical care was selected as an additional field for comparison because it is among the longest residency-plus-fellowship tracks at 7 years, and exemplifies the demands of combined clinical training. Finally, the triple board of pediatrics, adult psychiatry, and child and adolescent psychiatry was chosen as an example of combined training that includes psychiatric training.

Table 3-1 lists several medical specialties and the duration of training for each, and notes whether research activity and research literacy are required or encouraged by each specialty's RRC requirements. The table also lists the proportion of practicing physicians in each subspecialty who claim research as their primary activity, although these data have the obvious limitation of not characterizing those who engage in meaningful patient-oriented research on a more part-time basis. The final two columns of the table were determined by carefully reading the requirements of each specialty, identifying language concerning research education or direct research activity, and characterizing that language as mandatory or suggestive. In many cases, this determination was fairly straightforward, as the ACGME is explicit about the use of the terms "must" and "should." In other cases, the requirements are vague because, for example, "musts" are nested under "shoulds"; research activity is required for only some residents; or research activity is not differentiated from more generic endeavors such as "academic" activities or "scholarly pursuits." Despite these limitations, however, the table reflects whether research activity appears to be mandatory (a must) or suggested (a should) for most residents. The committee found no programs in which research is not mentioned, evidence that research content is considered one of the ingredients of medical education. The label of "should/must" is assigned to those descriptions that appear to fall between these designations (i.e., stronger than a "should", but not definitively a "must"). The triple board program (pediatrics, adult psychiatry, child and adolescent psychiatry) is assumed to conform to the ACGME requirements of its three parent specialties.

In addition to interviewing former Psychiatry RRC chairs, the committee carefully read the most recent RRC (2001) requirements for both adult (general) and child and adolescent psychiatry to understand as fully as possible the ACGME-mandated goals of residency training and to focus on the research training didactic learning or practical experiences included in those requirements. The first postgraduate year (PGY1) requires attainment of skills in history taking, diagnosis of mental and other medical disorders, continuous patient care, referrals, and doctor–patient communication. During PGY2 through PGY4, residents are "taught to conceptualize all illnesses in terms of biological, psychological, and sociocultural factors that determine normal and abnormal behavior" (ACGME, 2000b:Section V.A.2). Required clinical training includes "sufficient experiences" in the following: the diagnosis of disorders across a variety of age groups; short- and long-term psychotherapy, including psychodynamic therapy, group therapy, family therapy, and crisis intervention; drug detoxification; continuous care; psychiatric administration; neuropsychological testing; electroconvulsive therapy; and teaching (ACGME, 2000b:Section V.A.2.a). Child and adolescent psychiatrists are expected to master the same clinical concepts as adult trainees, with added emphasis on early brain and behavioral development.

TABLE 3-1 Summary of Duration, Time, and Research Requirements for Accredited Residency Training Programs in Selected Medical Specialties or Subspecialties

Specialty/ Subspecialty	Research Rates[a] (%)	Training Duration (months)	Time Allocations[b] (months)	Effective Date[c] (mo/yr)	Research Requirements[d] Activity[e]	Literacy[f]
Internal Medicine (general)	1.5	36	6 – Critical care 3 – Emergency 27 – Other int. med. Sub-specialties	7/2001	Must	Should
Allergy & Immunology	9.4	60	36 – Int. med. or pediatrics 6 – Research and scholarly activities 6 – Other educational activities 12 – Direct patient care	7/2002	Must	Must
Pulmonology/ Critical Care	1.0	72	36 – Int. med. 12 – Critical care (CC) 6 – Pulmonary disease (PD) 18 – CC/PD and other	7/1999	Must	Must
Pathology, Anatomic & Clinical	4.6	48	18 – Anatomic path (AP) 18 – Clinical path (CP) 12 – AP/CP or specialized training	7/2002	Should	Should

Specialty	%	Months	Breakdown	Date	Research	Research
Neurology	6.3	48	8 – Int. med./pediatrics; 18 – Adult neurology; 3 – Child neurology; 2 – Core sciences; 17 – Other	4/2002	Should/must	Must
Adult (General) Psychiatry	2.1	48	4 – Int. med./pediatrics/family med.; 2 – Neurology; 42 – Psychiatry	1/2001	Should/must	Should
Child & Adolescent Psychiatry	1.9	60	36 – Adult psychiatry; 24 – Child & adolescent psychiatry	1/2001	Should/must	Should/must
Triple Board[g]	N/A[h]	60	24 – Pediatrics; 36 – Adult and child & adolescent psychiatry	12/2001	N/A[h]	N/A[h]

---

[a] Proportion of physicians in specialty who claim research as their primary activity (same as used in Table 1-1).
[b] Vacation time not considered.
[c] Date when requirements were put into effect by the respective RRC, or the American Board of Psychiatry and Neurology for the triple board.
[d] Indicates whether written RRC requirements state that research activity by residents "must" or "should" be done, the former being a necessary component of training, the latter being an encouraged option of training.
[e] Refers to hands-on involvement in activities aimed at generating new medical knowledge.
[f] Refers to classroom teaching designed to give residents book knowledge about research concepts and methods.
[g] Assumed to conform to requirements of the 3 individual specialties: pediatrics, adult [general] psychiatry, child and adolescent psychiatry.
[h] N/A = not available.

SOURCE: Data obtained from AAMC (2002b), ABPN (2003a), ACGME (2002a), Pasko and Seidman (2002).

Boxes 3-1 and 3-2 summarize the clinical requirements for residents in adult psychiatry and child and adolescent psychiatry, respectively. A minimum of 31 months of the 4-year adult psychiatry program must be allocated to specific clinical training experiences (e.g., internal medicine, inpatient). Additionally, there are at least five untimed topic areas—emergency psychiatry, community psychiatry, forensic psychiatry, psychotherapies, and administration—that are covered in some form but can overlap with other, timed requirements (e.g., psychotherapy training can be covered in the context of inpatient or outpatient service). Untimed requirements not completed in the course of timed requirements must be completed in addition to the 31 months of timed training noted above. As mentioned earlier, the 5 years of child and adolescent psychiatry training typically encompasses 3 years of adult psychiatry followed by 2 years dedicated to child and adolescent training. These final 2 years include the clinical requirement of 4 to 10 months of service in a program that treats severely disabled children, but other requirements (of which there are at least six) are not timed.

Based on the information provided in Box 3-1, there appears to be a maximum of 13 months[15] of potential elective research time during the 4-year adult (general) psychiatry residency. Based on the information provided in Box 3-2, and assuming that the six untimed requirements in the box occupy 12 months of additional training time, child and adolescent psychiatry residents have a maximum of 8 months[16] of elective time. In reality, it appears that elective times are slightly below those figures, at approximately 8 months for adult and 4 months for child and adolescent training (see Appendix C for individual program summaries). Elective time for child training is especially constrained because the training combines two programs (i.e., adult and child) into just 12 months more than is allocated for adult training alone. Elective time is generally limited because the untimed requirements necessitate additional months of training, and because many programs choose or feel compelled by financial needs to maximize the service requirements of their residents to care for patients and generate clinical revenue (Miller, 2002). It should also be noted that among the constraints built into the training requirements is the fact the adult outpatient experience must be a *continuous* 12-month service. Despite these timed and untimed requirements, creative programs with the resources to overcome the loss of person-hours in the clinic or inpatient unit can offer 8- or 13-month electives to child and adult trainees, respectively, without violating the RRC re-

---

[15] This number assumes 1 month vacation per year of training.
[16] As with footnote 15.

quirements. Additionally, there are other opportunities to free up time for concentrated research training, as described in the next section.

BOX 3-1

Requirements Prescribed by the Psychiatry Residency Review Committee for Accredited Programs in Adult (General) Psychiatry

Topic	Required Duration (months)
Primary Care	4
Neurology	2
Outpatient	12^a
Inpatient	9 to 18^b
Child and Adolescent	2
Addiction	$(1)^c$
Geriatric	$(1)^c$
Consultation/Liaison	2^d
Emergency Psychiatry	NT^e
Community Psychiatry	NT^e
Forensic Psychiatry	NT^e
Psychotherapies	NT^e
Administrative	NT^e
Total Prescribed Time:	31 to 42^f

SOURCE: ACGME (2000b), Miller (2002).
[a] Must be a continuous service.
[b] Range is to place limits that yield minimal standards for training, but that prevent an institution from exploiting residents with excessive (i.e., >18 months) inpatient care responsibilities.
[c] This may be fulfilled as part of the inpatient or outpatient requirement
[d] One-month can be in pediatric consult/liaison.
[e] This requirement may take extra time to fulfill as it is not timed and does not necessarily overlap with a timed requirement.
[f] This figure does not account for mandatory vacation time, on the order of 1 month per year.

BOX 3-2

Requirements Prescribed by the Psychiatry Residency Review Committee for Accredited Programs in Child and Adolescent Psychiatry

Topic	Required Duration (months)
Adult (general) psychiatry	31 to 42 (see Box 3-1)
Experience with acutely and severely disabled children and adolescents in an organized treatment program	4 to 10[a]
Evaluation, treatment of "sufficient numbers of children and adolescents with a broad range of psychiatric illness"	NT[b]
Psychotherapies in children and adolescents	NT[b]
Supervised collaboration with other professional mental health practitioners	NT[b]
Psychological testing	NT[b]
Pediatric neurology	NT[b]
Consult role to children, adolescents, and their families	NT[b]
Total Prescribed Time:	35 to 52[c]

SOURCE: ACGME (2000a)

[a] Range is to place limits that yield minimal standards for training, but that prevent an institution from exploiting residents with excessive (i.e., >10 months) patient care responsibilities.

[b] This requirement may take extra time to fulfill as it is not timed and will not likely overlap with the one timed requirement noted.

[c] This figure does not account for mandatory vacation time, on the order of 1 month per year.

Other Opportunities for Research Experiences in Residency

There are a number of opportunities to shorten some of the clinical requirements mandated by the Psychiatry RRC. First, some of the requirements—consultation/liaison (2 months), addiction (1 month), and geriatric psychiatry (1 month)—are potentially redundant. Each of these psychiatric subspecialties might alternatively be covered during inpatient and outpatient clinical service, and in fact the latter two can be covered during those rotations. Consultation/liaison could be part of inpatient or outpatient service if the organizational infrastructure existed to divide residents' time between direct patient care and periodic outside contacts. Addiction and geriatric subspecialty clinical encounters can be part of the normal practice of inpatient and outpatient psychiatric care. Given the high rate of comorbidity of various psychiatric illnesses and substance abuse disorders, it is probable that in many clinics, psychiatric residents will have ample opportunity to treat the latter disorders (Chen et al., 1992; Regier et al., 1990). Similarly, frequent contact with elderly patients at some facilities may offer sufficient exposure to geriatric practice without a separate rotation.

Second, the inpatient requirements may be too long, and not in accordance with recent trends in medical care. As is the case with all branches of medicine, the length of inpatient stays has decreased dramatically in psychiatry (Eisenberg, 2002; Henderson, 2000; Mechanic, 1998; Pottick et al., 2000; Sturm and Bao, 2000), thereby making outpatient and community-based interventions increasingly relevant to long-term outcomes. As hospital stays have shortened, residents' experiences in inpatient services have increasingly become limited to the three early phases of a disease episode: diagnosis, stabilization, and discharge. Absent from those experiences are the important phases of recovery and maintenance, two aspects of treatment that are of obvious importance to the patient, and that can also be extremely gratifying to a training psychiatrist and a potential patient-oriented psychiatrist-researcher. Accordingly, the 9-month inpatient service that is prescribed by the adult requirements might be reduced to accommodate programs having the infrastructure to engage their residents in greater outpatient care or even in patient-oriented research activities.

Third, the psychotherapy requirements are excessive in their expectations, and some lack a sufficient evidence-base. According to these requirements, "The program must demonstrate that residents have achieved competency in at least the following forms of psychotherapy: brief therapy, cognitive behavioral therapy, combined psychotherapy and psychopharmacology, psychodynamic therapy, and supportive therapy"

(ACGME, 2000b:Section VI.B.2). As discussed earlier in this chapter, psychodynamics is particularly problematic because there have been few if any clinical trials supporting the efficacy of this therapy (Eisenberg, 2002), although some findings may be emerging (Simpson et al., 2003). Additionally, it appears unrealistic that, during a 4- or 5-year residency crowded with numerous other responsibilities and learning requirements, residents can achieve competency in all of these different forms of psychotherapy; this is true especially for psychodynamics, given its complexity and typical duration. As an alternative, the committee suggests that the psychotherapy requirement be modified to mandate more generic attainment of competency in psychotherapy while offering the option for competency achievement in specific forms such as psychodynamics. The aim should be to train psychiatrists in evidence-based psychotherapy methods and provide them with sophisticated knowledge common to all major forms of psychotherapy.

As a possible guide to such training goals, Beitman and Yue (1999) detail a curriculum consolidating common factors that cut across various psychotherapeutic approaches. This curriculum parses psychotherapy into the generic and chronological stages of (1) engagement, (2) pattern search, (3) change, and (4) termination. This parsing of general constructs is used to teach trainees psychotherapeutic concepts and skills that can be adapted to a variety of clinical situations. It also gives trainees theoretical connectivity to many of the major schools of psychotherapy, including psychodynamics. Along with such didactic training, the RRC requirements could mandate that residents become competent in a small number (e.g., two) of distinct evidence-based psychotherapies. The precise choice of methods could be left to the individual training program and also to the personal, albeit monitored, goals of the trainees themselves. This 'pick list' approach is not the committee's idea, but one that was suggested during the last revision of the Psychiatry RRC requirements (personal communication, D. Winstead, Tulane University, April 7, 2003). To the extent that certain programs wish to offer more extended psychotherapy training of any type, 1-year fellowships, similar to those currently in existence for substance abuse, pain management, and forensics, could be created to train a subset of psychiatrists (ACGME, 1995a; 1995b; 1996). As stated previously in this chapter, emphasis of evidence-based methods in the training of psychiatrists has the potential added benefit of attracting research-oriented medical students who may have been discouraged by psychiatry's apparent over-reliance on traditional practice methods.

A fourth opportunity to expand research training time lies in the fact that the RRC clinical requirements unnecessarily constrain the schedule of child and adolescent psychiatry trainees because they must fulfill many of the same service requirements as adult psychiatrists. Thus they are prevented from following the obvious path of focusing more on pediatric medicine from the outset of their residency. Part of the issue is that some residents do not choose to enter the child and adolescent subspecialty until they have already completed much of their adult training, which is the foundation of the specialty, whereas some make the choice early enough that they might exchange some adult service time for more time in child and adolescent service. Accordingly, for psychiatric trainees who commit to child and adolescent training early (PGY1), the following types of adjustments to the training requirements might logically be permissible and act as an incentive to pursue a specialty that currently is in great need of more applicants (Kim et al., 2001): 2 months of adult neurology could be exchanged for pediatric neurology (an untimed requirement); 12 months of adult outpatient service could be reduced and replaced by requirements associated with child outpatient service; the substance abuse requirements could be focused on those issues in childhood and adolescence; and the geriatrics requirement could be eliminated from child and adolescent training or folded into adult inpatient training as suggested previously in this report for general psychiatric trainees.

Overall, careful consideration of the need for various timed requirements is consistent with the ACGME's Outcome Project. This project has already developed a list of six general competencies for all physicians: patient care, medical knowledge, practice-based learning and improvement, interpersonal and communication skills, professionalism, and system-based practice. The overall aim is to emphasize product (e.g., educational outcome) over process (e.g., timed requirements, number of patients seen) to further the goal of efficient preparation of medical residents (ACGME, 2002b; Batalden et al., 2002). The committee strongly supports this approach, and believes it has the potential to provide programs with the flexibility to reward qualified and motivated residents with earlier and more extensive research training.

Research Requirements for Psychiatric Residency

A recent survey of 70 research-oriented departments of psychiatry among 126 allopathic U.S. and Canadian medical schools revealed that although 91 percent of these departments reported having a research didactic in their residency programs, only 28 percent of those programs offered instruction in research design. The aggregate amount of time these programs spent on research topics generally was less than 6 percent of the total curriculum (Balon and Singh, 2001).

To investigate this apparent dearth of research training time, the committee reviewed the research requirements of the Psychiatry RRC in both adult and child and adolescent psychiatry and compared them with the requirements for several other medical specialties (see Table 3-1 above for a summary of clinical and research requirements of various programs). With regard to these requirements, the Psychiatry RRC uses what appears to be "boilerplate" language, similar to that appearing in the written requirements of other medical specialties. The requirements of the Psychiatry RRC state that residency training "must" take place in an "environment of inquiry and scholarship in which residents participate in the development of new knowledge" and "should" include such scholarly activities as journal clubs, conferences, peer-reviewed publications, and research projects, as well as "guidance and technical support for resident participation in scholarly activities." Pathology and neurology have similarly worded requirements. However, the Pathology RRC emphasizes these requirements in a separate section titled "Resident Research," which explicitly calls for the encouragement and promotion of resident involvement in research activities, while the Neurology RRC appears to mandate research literacy for all residents to a greater extent than is the case for either pathology or psychiatry. It appears, then, that both pathology and neurology have slightly stronger written expectations for research training during residency as compared with psychiatry, although the differences among the three sets of requirements are small.

A&I and subspecialties of internal medicine (e.g., pulmonology/critical care), on the other hand, have much more explicit requirements. The foundation of A&I training is 3 years of internal medicine or pediatrics residency, followed by 2 years focused on specialty training. During these last 2 years of training, the A&I requirements specifically state that accredited programs must provide documentation that "each resident" engages in at least 25 percent time "devoted to research and scholarly activities." Stronger still are the requirements for subspecialties of internal medicine, which state:

> As part of the academic environment, an active research component must be included within each accredited subspecialty program. The program must ensure a meaningful, supervised research experience with appropriate protected time—either in blocks or concurrent with clinical rotations—for each resident, while maintaining the essential clinical experience. Evidence of recent productiv-

ity by both the program faculty and by the residents as a whole, will be required, including publication in peer-reviewed journals. Residents must learn the design and interpretation of research studies, responsible use of informed consent, and research methodology and interpretation of data. The program must provide instruction in the critical assessment of new therapies and of the medical literature. Residents should be advised and supervised by qualified faculty members in the conduct of research. (ACGME, 1999:Section V.L)

The impact of these strong requirements may be related to the higher rates of research involvement by allergists/immunologists (9.8 percent) and by subspecialists of internal medicine (about 6 percent) compared with those seen among psychiatrists (2 percent; see Table 3-1). It is notable, however, that those who undergo the combined training for pulmonology/critical care appear to opt for research careers in the lowest proportion, so the requirement alone does not guarantee later involvement. Nevertheless, to the extent that the field of psychiatry wants to increase their profession's involvement in research, the Psychiatry RRC should follow the examples set by A&I and subspecialties of internal medicine with regard to both research participation and, at a minimum, research literacy[17] requirements for their residents and residency curricula. As they stand now, the psychiatry requirements are confusing and sometimes ambiguous. For example, "musts" are nested under "shoulds." An example is the requirement (ACGME, 2000b:Section V.D.1.a) that the "following components of a scholarly environment *should* be present...the program *must* promote an atmosphere of scholarly inquiry, including the provision of access to ongoing research activity...[emphasis added]." Stated another way, it appears that some requirements are actually optional, a situation that could confuse program administrators about the level of resources they need to devote to research training, didactic or otherwise.

---

[17] Research literacy is the ability to interpret existing and emerging scientific information critically and adapt or reject that information for the ongoing practice of quality medical care. The term further refers to an understanding of the effort that goes into developing new medical knowledge.

CERTIFICATION BOARD, AMERICAN BOARD OF PSYCHIATRY AND NEUROLOGY

As noted earlier, the ABPN is one of three groups that appoint members to the Psychiatry RRC. The ABPN is responsible for five appointments (three ABPN directors and two child and adolescent psychiatrists) to the Psychiatry RRC and has input into the process for formulating program requirements. In contrast with the Psychiatry RRC, which accredits residency training *programs*, the ABPN certifies *individual psychiatrists* by means of written and oral examinations and an audit of specific training experiences leading up to those examinations (ABPN, 2003b). The ABPN examination focuses primarily on direct patient care issues in which certified clinicians should be proficient (see Box 3-3). There are virtually no questions devoted to research methodology and data analysis, with the possible exception of a few questions on statistics in the epidemiology section and on experimental psychology approaches in the behavioral and social sciences section.

As of April 2003, the ABPN had no official policies regarding research training during residency and had not implemented or suggested training pathways that would support research in residency (personal communication, S. Scheiber, ABPN, April 3, 2003). Although most other specialty boards also lack research tracks, the dermatology, anesthesiology, pediatrics, and internal medicine boards, at least, have developed such pathways (Hostetter, 2002; IOM, 1994). The pediatrics and internal medicine pathways are described in Chapter 2. The dermatology training track is similar to the regular track that includes basic or clinical research training for all residents, but the research track allows the explicit integration (in lieu of other training activities) of investigative or didactic experience after PGY2 has been completed (American Board of Dermatology, 2003). The anesthesiology pathway has two options: option A involves 6 months of clinical or basic research in the context of a 48-month residency; option B involves 18 months of research in the context of a 60-month residency (The American Board of Anesthesiology, 2002).

The ABPN has considerable influence on residency-based research training in at least three ways. First, as noted above, the ABPN appoints one-third of the membership to the Psychiatry RRC. Second, it must approve all applicants for the certification examination, and this approval process involves retrospective determination of whether a given applicant completed all the prescribed RRC requirements (e.g., months of clinical service). Third, the ABPN is responsible for the content of the certification examination, thereby encouraging residents to learn certain facts and concepts in lieu of others (ABPN, 2002). Thus it is arguably the principal national organizing body that can impact residency training, and residency-based research training efforts that are not in some fashion sanctioned or promoted by the ABPN are likely to have more limited success than those that are.

BOX 3-3

Summary of Topics Included on Written Portion of Psychiatry Board Examination

Topic	Number of Questions
Psychiatry Content (total 260 questions)	
Psychiatric disorders	78
Treatments	78
Neuroscienes	26
Diagnostic procedures	23
Brain and psychosocial development through the life cycle	16
Behavioral and social sciences	13
Epidemiology and public policy	13
Special topics (e.g., suicide, emergency psychiatry)	13
Neurology Content (total 160 questions)	
Clinical evaluation	56
Basic science of neurologic disorders	32
Diagnostic procedures	32
Management and treatment	32
Incidence risk	8
Total number of questions on Part I examination	420

NOTE: The approximate number of questions devoted to each topic area was calculated from content percentages specified in outline form at the ABPN website.
SOURCE: ABPN (2002).

AMERICAN MEDICAL ASSOCIATION

The AMA Council on Medical Education (CME) nominates six (five voting, one ex officio) members to the Psychiatry RRC. Although experience in graduate medical education is a very important selection factor, research experience is not necessarily considered relevant (personal communication, B. Barzansky, AMA, October 22, 2002). In its 2002 annual report to the AMA membership, the CME commented about a great variety of issues affecting graduate medical education, including resident work hours, Medicare funding for graduate medical education, and medical school debt. Research training was not explicitly mentioned in this report, although the importance of continuous evaluation of best practices in medical education was a clearly stated goal (CME, 2003). Given the importance of training clinical scientists to develop and validate contemporary best practices, one can only assume that the AMA would support efforts to enhance research training in the psychiatric residency.

OTHER NATIONAL ORGANIZATIONS INVOLVED IN PSYCHIATRIC RESEARCH TRAINING

American Psychiatric Association

In addition to the ABPN and the AMA, professional societies for psychiatrists have addressed and fostered research training. The APA is the largest, with nearly 40,000 members (APA, 2002b). Its Division of Education, Minority, and National Programs nominates directors to the ABPN, and also appoints six members (five full, one liaison) to the Psychiatry RRC. The APA also operates the American Psychiatric Institute for Research and Education (APIRE) and the Council on Research (COR), which administer educational, lobbying, and research training activities that promote and develop mental health research and awareness at the national level. As described in Chapter 2, APIRE and the COR manage several research fellowships. The COR has created an annual Research Colloquium for Junior Investigators, which is timed to coincide with the annual APA meeting. Started in 1996, the program provides 45 awards (of $1000 each) annually to senior residents, fellows, and junior faculty to attend a 1-day meeting. At that meeting, they discuss their research goals with peers and senior psychiatric researchers, who offer advice and guidance regarding a research career (APA, 2003). A retrospective study of participants in the colloquia from 1996 to 1999 found that 114 of the 118 respondents reported some continued degree of research involvement since participating (APA 2002c). Of that group, 67 had received local department research funding, and 80 had received external funding, including 35 federal grants, as principal investigators (APA 2002c). Although these data cannot be used to assess the impact of the colloquia, they do suggest that the program is succeeding in bringing together a good number of newly developing psychiatrist-researchers.

American Academy of Child and Adolescent Psychiatry

The American Academy of Child and Adolescent Psychiatry (AACAP) is a professional society of child and adolescent psychiatrists with more than 6,000 members. Unlike the APA, the AACAP does not have the authority to appoint members to the Psychiatry RRC. However, it does have several small-scale research training initiatives. These initiatives, funded by the federal government and pharmaceutical companies, provide fellowship (see Chapter 2 for more detail) or seminar experiences (AACAP, 2002a; 2002c; 2002d). Somewhat analogous to the APA colloquia, the Early Investigators Group (EIG) was initiated by the AACAP in 2000 to facilitate the development of new researchers by providing a venue for professional networking and informal peer review (AACAP, 2003a). The AACAP has also convened a task force to develop a residency-based curriculum aimed at training child psychiatrist-researchers and one that that also integrates research content throughout the residency (i.e., beginning in PGY1 and continuing through the final year) (see the description in Chapter 4) (personal communication, J. Leckman, Yale University, April 4, 2003[18]). Key features of this curriculum are an emphasis on core competencies that include "research skills," and opportunities for outstanding students to accelerate their training to permit increased time for hands-on research over the course of a 5- or 6-year residency training period.

---

[18] Communication via the following document: Version 5.0 (February 2003) of *Integrated Residency Training in Child and Adolescent and Adult Psychiatry*, a product of a task force assembled by the AACAP.

Other National Organizations

Other national organizations relevant to psychiatric practice and research training include, but are not limited to, the American Association of Directors of Psychiatry Residency Training (AADPRT), the American Association of Chairs of Departments of Psychiatry (AACDP), the Association of Directors of Medical Student Education in Psychiatry (ADMSEP), and the American College of Neuropsychopharmacology (ACNP). These organizations represent the perspectives of residency training directors, department chairs, student clerkship directors, and psychopharmacologists, respectively. None of them has a direct impact (i.e., nominating or voting rights) on the Psychiatry RRC or the ABPN. Nevertheless, some organizations, such as the AADPRT, may have an impact on RRC requirements, as AADPRT members are asked to comment on new RRC requirements before these requirements are finalized.[19] Moreover, these organizations interact regularly with RRC representatives at meetings and in the context of ongoing program accreditation and review processes. Over the course of this report, it became clear to the committee that all of these organizations have at least some appreciation for the importance of research and research training opportunities in the context of psychiatric residency, although many tend to be focused on more immediate, day-to-day clinical training and practice issues.

CONCLUSIONS AND RECOMMENDATIONS

The two regulatory bodies with the greatest influence over residency training are the Psychiatry RRC and the ABPN. The committee understands and respects the fact that these two bodies aim to safeguard consumer health by ensuring that residency graduates are trained to deliver quality psychiatric care. We also understand that a national regulatory effort is complex and that defined requirements (both timed and untimed) are useful in the documentation of residency training. At the same time, the committee believes the requirements are so expansive and prescriptive that they impair the development of timely research training experiences for residents; and requirements currently exist that are redundant or do not represent the best available evidence-based practices in psychiatry. Given the apparent excessive nature of the requirements and the universal belief that protected time for research activity is critical for re-

---

[19] A public comment period is part of the formal approval process used by all ACGME committees.

search success (Costa et al., 2000; DeHaven et al., 1998; Griggs, 2002; McGuire and Fairbanks, 1982; Raphael et al., 1990; Roberts and Bogenschutz, 2001; Schrier, 1997; Shine, 1998; Shore et al., 2001), the committee makes the following recommendation:

> **Recommendation 3.1. The American Board of Psychiatry and Neurology and the Psychiatry Residency Review Committee should make the requirements for board certification and residency accreditation more flexible so research training can occur during residency at a level that significantly increases the probability of more residents choosing research as a career. The committee further recommends that residents who successfully fulfill core requirements at an accelerated pace, with competency being used as the measure, be allowed to spend the time thus made available to pursue research training.**

This recommendation is aimed at optimizing core training by minimizing redundant and non–evidence-based aspects of that training, and by giving programs and individuals the opportunity to tailor larger portions of their training to incorporate elective experiences that might include hands-on research activity. The recommendation further aims to entice outstanding residents to undertake research activity by rewarding fast-paced attainment of clinical competency with greater opportunities for early research involvement. Implementation of this recommendation will depend on clear guidelines from both the RRC and the ABPN. This guidance might be delivered most efficiently if the RRC and the ABPN jointly published a clearly defined checklist for use by training directors and residents in determining what requirements and electives must be fulfilled for accreditation and certification. Implementation of this recommendation will also depend upon the development of criteria for determining when and whether a resident has developed a level of competency that warrants special advancement into an accelerate research track. Although the development of such criteria poses logistic challenges for training programs, existing instruments, such as the Psychiatry Resident In-Training Examination (PRITE), could be used along with supervisor evaluations to certify accelerated resident competency (American College of Psychiatrists, 2002).

At the same time that the committee advocates increased flexibility in clinical requirements, we also believe that the research requirements of residency training must be strengthened if the field of psychiatry is to keep pace in the age of evidence-based medical practice. Although the RRC requirements do offer research experiences and didactic learning as clear "shoulds," most programs appear to offer very limited research training to their residents (Balon and Singh, 2001), and even the strongest programs delay research experiences until late in the residency (see Chapter 4). Accordingly, the committee makes the following recommendation:

> **Recommendation 3.2. The American Board of Psychiatry and Neurology and the Psychiatry Residency Review Committee should require patient-oriented research literacy as a core competency of residency training in adult and child and adolescent psychiatry. Program directors and the American Board of Psychiatry and Neurology should evaluate residents on these competencies.**

Both the ABPN and the Psychiatry RRC must recognize that patient-oriented research and patient care are inextricably linked. This should include accreditation and credentialing requirements that make research literacy essential and research experiences desirable goals of all residency programs toward the aim of training clinicians who will be capable of incorporating the latest knowledge into their practice. Gaining research experience in addition to literacy is important for two reasons: first, research experiences contribute to literacy by allowing residents to understand the challenges and details of research activity; second, the opportunity to engage in research work may convince some residents of their unique talent for or interest in such activity. Recommendation 3.2 should be implemented by strengthening the language in the Psychiatry RRC requirements to indicate that all residents should be familiar with research design and methods such that they are prepared for the lifelong practice of evidence-based medicine. As currently written, the requirements for research training are ambiguous: on the one hand, they say "a program *must* promote an atmosphere of scholarly inquiry including the provision of ongoing research activity in psychiatry [emphasis added]," but on the other hand, they say that the "didactic curriculum *should* include...research methods in the clinical and behavioral sciences related to psychiatry [emphasis added]."

The ABPN could further enforce the literacy requirement by adding more questions on the certification examination designed to explicitly test research literacy. Content for the examination and for program didactics in the context of residency training could come from any number of works on clinical research in psychiatry or other branches of medicine, works that could also be used to design research literacy curricula. Blazer and Hays (1998), for example, crafted a text that uses real-world, peer-reviewed examples to teach readers the concepts and shortcomings of scientific inference, study design, and analysis and interpretation as these concepts pertain to clinical research in psychiatry. The next chapter describes several other curricula in clinical research.

To best develop these competencies and also optimally integrate research training into residency training, the involvement of researchers in the full educational development process will be important. Thus, the following recommendation is made:

Recommendation 3.3. The organizations that nominate members for the Psychiatry Residency Review Committee and the American Board of Psychiatry and Neurology should include on their nomination lists substantial numbers of extramurally funded, experienced psychiatrist-investigators who conduct patient-oriented research.

As discussed above, research experience is not currently an explicit requirement for nomination to the Psychiatry RRC or to the ABPN, yet there is concern among both regulatory bodies and among researchers themselves that experienced researchers are not sufficiently involved in the formal expectation-setting process for residents. It is the committee's view that at least some of the slots on those regulatory bodies should be filled with individuals who are skilled as patient-oriented researchers. Their involvement would greatly increase the probability that accreditation and certification policies will be influenced by those with first-hand knowledge of what a career in patient-oriented research requires. Implementation of recommendation 3.3 could be undertaken by one of the nominating bodies (e.g., APA, AMA) or through a change in the written nomination policies of the ACGME and the ABPN to mandate the inclusion of a certain number of patient-oriented researchers.

Implementation of this recommendation will obviously be limited by the relatively small number of researchers in the field. Therefore, researchers themselves should be prepared to sacrifice some time to contibute to the educational mission, while others in psychiatry should consider how to make these service responsibilities tenable to those who might prefer to be otherwise engaged. For example, service on the ABPN executive board requires a commitment of 45 days per year (personal communication, S. Scheiber, ABPN, April 3, 2003). For those with a sizable research program, a 45-day (or even a much shorter) commitment may be impossible unless their department chair or extramural funding agency offers them some reprieve or extension on existing obligations (e.g., a no-cost extension, supplemental support). As an alternative to full committee service, such researchers could be called upon to serve on subcommittees or in other more limited capacities. Regardless of the form it takes, the goal of such researcher involvement in ABPN and RRC affairs should be for experienced patient-oriented researchers to have a genuine and measurable impact on the requirements and priorities established each year by these regulatory bodies. Compromise on the part of those who have traditionally served on these bodies and a sacrifice of time by researchers who have sometimes avoided such service will both be necessary if this recommendation is to be implemented.

Although this chapter focuses on regulatory issues, which in this case involve the oversight of the Psychiatry RRC and the ABPN, these bodies do not act in a vacuum. A number of other national stakeholders (e.g., the AADPRT, APA, and AACAP) have an interest in residency training, although their approach appears typically to consist of offering small initiatives, such as 1-day seminars, or targeting postresidency trainees for research support in the context of fellowships (see above and Chapter 2). Nevertheless, these efforts appear to be focused sincerely on increasing research training in psychiatry, including the residency context. A notable example is the AACAP's recent initiative to develop and broadly disseminate a model curriculum for child and adolescent psychiatry residency programs interested in infusing more research into their training curriculum. This initiative, though spearheaded by the AACAP, was undertaken with the cooperation of both the RRC and the ABPN (personal communication, J. Leckman, Yale University, April 4, 2003; personal communication, S. Scheiber, ABPN, April 3, 2003). These efforts indicate that a national consensus is emerging with regard to the importance of residency-based research training; Chapter 6 addresses the importance of harnessing that emerging consensus to further the cause.

Finally, it should be noted that regulatory guidance and constraints on programs do not act in isolation. The policies of the Psychiatry RRC and the ABPN clearly set values for the entire field, but these organizations do not directly train residents to be researchers. Local institutions need to provide resources and opportunities, including research time, mentors, and a culture that genuinely values the importance of generating new clinical knowledge. The next chapter details the state of research training at the institutional level.

4

Institutional Factors

The last chapter focused on regulatory issues that influence psychiatric research training during residency, noting that national oversight of the residency accreditation and board certification processes has considerable influence on the goals of residency training, research literacy, and research training. This chapter looks more directly at the programs themselves, considering the obstacles and strategies of institutions and departments regarding research training during residency. As financial constraints are central to this subject, the chapter begins with a brief discussion of how residency education is typically funded in the United States. It then addresses two key institutional factors that influence research training during residency: leadership and mentoring, and program and curriculum structure. The chapter ends with conclusions and recommendations that include a theoretical framework for evaluating institutions that aim to offer research education to psychiatry trainees.

FUNDING ISSUES IN GRADUATE MEDICAL EDUCATION

The General Funding Stream

Graduate medical education (GME) funding for all residents comes primarily from the following sources: Medicare, Medicaid, the Veterans Administration, the Department of Defense, the National Institutes of Health (NIH), and the private sector (see Table 4-1) (Anderson et al.,

2001). As the numbers in Table 4-1 indicate, Medicare is the largest single source of GME funding. Medicare is also currently the most reliable source of GME funding because federal law requires annual entitlement payments to institutions that serve Medicare patients to subsidize both "direct" and "indirect" costs associated with training new physicians. Direct medical education (DME) payments subsidize resident stipends and benefits, faculty teaching time, and educational infrastructure. Indirect medical education (IME) payments, which are nearly twice as large as DME, are designed to subsidize the less visible costs associated with GME, including the fact that trainees tend to deliver less efficient care than do more experienced physicians (e.g., overprescribing tests), and that teaching hospitals typically treat the most severely ill patients. In an effort to minimize short-term operating costs, nongovernmental third-party payers are inclined to avoid GME costs that do not relate directly to patient care (e.g., certain IME costs or stipends for residents doing research training) (Knapp, 2002). This inclination has placed general financial pressure on the educational mission of institutions that train residents. It has also led to the introduction of proposed federal legislation aimed at ensuring that all users of medical care contribute equally to GME funding—legislation that was originally introduced by the late Senator Moynihan (D-NY) in 1999 and that has the strong support of the Association of American Medical Colleges (AAMC, 2001).

TABLE 4-1 Sources of Graduate Medical Education Funding

Source	Amount (billions of dollars)
Medicare	7.8^a (2.7 direct, 5.1 indirect)
Medicaid	2.3^b
VA/DOD/NIH^c	2.0^d
Private-Sector Payers	6.0

NOTES:
^{a}Year: 2000.
^{b}Year: 1998.
^{c}Veterans Administration/Department of Defense/National Institutes of Health.
^{d}In 2001, NIH training grants and fellowships accounted for $300 million of this amount. As these training and fellowship grants include Ph.D.'s and medical residents, the NIH contribution to GME is well below that $300 million dollar amount.
SOURCE: Anderson et al. (2001).

Funding Issues in Pediatric Graduate Medical Education

Institutions that treat predominantly pediatric populations may receive lower amounts of GME funding than other institutions because they are less likely to treat Medicare's primary beneficiary—the elderly. As a result, they are dependent upon non-Medicare sources, which are not entitlements and are subject to annual local or federal appropriations processes (Henderson, 2000).[20] Although child and adolescent psychiatry residents at Medicare-funded institutions are considered 100 percent full-time equivalents (FTEs) for reimbursement calculation purposes, the reimbursement is based on an institution's Medicare utilization, an index that reduces the reimbursement rate for institutions with a high pediatric caseload. Additionally, in child and adolescent psychiatry, as with all Accreditation Council for Graduate Medical Education (ACGME)-designated *sub*specialties, GME coverage drops to 50 percent for each FTE in postgraduate year 5 (PGY5) (ACGME, 2000a) because the Medicare law offers full reimbursement only for what the ACGME defines as "general" training (American Academy of Child and Adolescent Psychiatry [AACAP], 2002b).[21] It is notable that child and adolescent psychiatry is considered a subspecialty of adult (general) psychiatry, even though pediatrics is not considered a subspecialty of internal medicine.

Supporting Research Activity Through Graduate Medical Education Funds

Research training is peripheral to immediate clinical care. Consequently, there are some limits on the use of Medicare GME funding to cover residents engaged in research training activities. A review of federal regulations pertaining to GME reimbursement from Medicare indicates that neither DME nor IME reimbursements are intended to cover activities outside of patient care.[21,22,23] One regulation explicitly states: "The time spent by a resident in research that is not associated with the treatment or diagnosis of a particular patient is not countable."[22] This regulation clearly excludes "basic research" on nonhumans, although it

---

[20] Healthcare Research and Quality Act of 1999. Pub. L. No. 106-129 (1999); Children's Health Act of 2000. Pub. L. No. 106-310 (2000).

[21] Direct Graduate Medical Education Payments. 42 C.F.R. §413.86 (2001).

[22] Special treatment: Hospitals that incur indirect costs for graduate medical education programs. 42 C.F.R. §412.105 (1999).

[23] HHS (Health and Human Services). Counting Research Time as Direct and Indirect GME Costs. F.R.66(148): 39896. 2001.

does not necessarily limit patient-oriented research, especially if such activity involves regular patient contact.

Since the federal regulations additionally defer to the ACGME for determining the legitimacy of reimbursable resident activities, there is room for educational activities not exclusively linked to billable clinical productivity. Nevertheless, the concern that funding may be reduced if residents engage in research training adds uncertainty to an already tenuous stream of federal support for residency training in general. This concern prompted officials at the University of Michigan to obtain a grant from the National Institute of Mental Health (NIMH) to cover their psychiatry residency-based research training program (McCullum-Smith, 2002). Concern has also been heightened in the New England area as that region's Medicare intermediary has asked institutions to refund GME money that supported residents engaged in "bench" research. Although the action targeted surgery residency programs that permitted a full "year-out" for residents to conduct basic laboratory work, it has had a discouraging effect on residency-based research training initiatives more broadly, especially those that involve basic research training components (personal communication, S. Benjamin, University of Massachusetts Medical School, July 22, 2002).

The committee validated the above described Medicare restrictions on research activity by interviewing GME directors at institutions in Arizona, Arkansas, Georgia, and Washington State. These GME directors verified that research, and especially basic research activity by residents, typically is not reimbursable by Medicare. They also indicated that increased scrutiny by Medicare intermediaries is part of a more general effort among third-party payers to control their costs. At the same time, these GME directors were all aware that clinical research activities that encompass the diagnosis and treatment of patients are reimbursable under Medicare, although they acknowledged that the regulations are sometimes confusing to those engaged in the accounting process.

A further and important consideration is the institutional flow of GME dollars. These funds usually are directed to hospitals rather than to departmental residency programs, and federal legislation dating back to 1986 prevents expanding the numbers of medical residents funded by Medicare (Knapp, 2002).[24] Given the variability in institutional and departmental needs, GME funding for psychiatry training programs may or may not be proportional to the size of those programs. Training slots may be reallocated to other departments, or IME dollars, which are tendered by an institution to support the general training environment, may not

---

[24] Consolidated Omnibus Budget Reconciliation Act of 1985, Pub. L. No. 97-272 (1986).

proportionally finance all departments responsible for training residents. Thus, the flow of funds to support residency and fellowship training may be more generous for one program than another, adding to the uncertainty faced by individual training programs regarding their operating budgets.

It is unclear whether GME funding adequately covers the true cost of training the next generation of medical doctors. What is known, however, is that resident compensation is far below what entry-level physicians earn after graduating from residency—a reality that has prompted some analysts to argue that residents themselves bear considerable cost in the training endeavor (Newhouse and Wilensky, 2001), and that furthermore is tied to a recent lawsuit by 200,000 medical residents claiming that the GME matching system supports the economic exploitation of physician trainees (AAMC, 2003; Miller and Greaney, 2003).

Additionally, cost-saving measures in recent years have eroded general GME funding streams to teaching hospitals, as well as direct and indirect streams of capital to research training. Moreover, residency funding for pediatric programs, including child and adolescent psychiatry programs, is currently even less secure than funding for programs involving a substantial Medicare patient load.

The above are key financial realities faced by all U.S. residency training programs, including those that train psychiatrists.

General Research Funding

Layered over the GME funding constraints described above are the general financial challenges imposed by the emergence of managed care. Across all of medicine, clinical reimbursement rates have decreased, yielding lower per-hour incomes for individual physicians and for the departments in which they serve. As a result of lower clinical incomes, residents and faculty have less discretionary time for research and research mentoring because they need to increase clinical volume to compensate for the lower reimbursement rates (AAMC, 2002b; Beresin, 1997; Ludmerer, 1999; Mirin, 2002; Pardes, 2002). Additionally, lower clinical income reduces the surplus revenues traditionally used by institutions to cross-subsidize research and other activities not encompassed by the clinical mission (AAMC, 1999; Jones and Sanderson, 1996). A recent study by the Commonwealth Fund Taskforce on Academic Health Centers (1999) found that nearly 10 percent of research at academic health centers is supported by surplus from faculty practice plans. Perhaps even more important, Moy et al. (1997) found that managed care penetration not only decreases surpluses from clinical work, but also appears to discourage institutions from seeking federal research dollars. This finding is particularly important as federal grants account for nearly 70 percent of the research funding for academic health centers (Commonwealth Fund Taskforce on Academic Health Centers, 1999).

For departments of psychiatry, shortages in clinical income may be even more acute. Despite the recent introduction of mental health parity laws that have required some insurers to cover mental disorders at levels similar to those for other diseases, full mental health care coverage remains patchy both geographically (i.e., state by state) and with regard to the extent of coverage (e.g., small employers have been exempt from federal provisions, and parity for addiction is often excluded) (Frank et al., 2001b). Recent estimates cited in the Surgeon General's Report on Mental Health indicate that as of 1997, medium to large corporations were offering mental health benefits to their employees valued at 3 percent of the total medical benefits, down from 6 percent just 10 years earlier (DHHS, 1999; HayGroup, 1999). Given the increased awareness of mental disorders and treatment that occurred during this decade (see Chapter 1) and the Surgeon General's estimate that mental disorders account for more than 15 percent of the disease burden in industrialized countries, a 3 percent insurance benefit appears disproportionately low. Another analysis reported by the Surgeon General determined that if a family experienced $35,000 in mental health expenses during a given year, that family would be responsible for $12,000 out of pocket, compared with only $1,500 in out-of-pocket expenses for equally costly medical/surgical care in the same year (Zuvekas et al., 1998). This lack of insurance/reimbursement equity adds to the financial pressure faced by psychiatrists and other mental health practitioners with regard to declining clinical revenues secondary to managed care, and diminishes the opportunity to partially fund clinical research from patient care revenues.

These financial realities exist in an age when patient-oriented research costs are increasing as a result of the growing complexity of such investigative endeavors (AAMC, 1999). Psychiatric research, like other biomedical research, relies on a multidisciplinary team approach (Beresin, 1997; Institute of Medicine [IOM], 2000; Meador-Woodruff, 2002; Meyer and McLaughlin, 1998; Roberts and Bogenschutz, 2001). For example, a brain imaging study of psychiatric patients requires not only considerable material investment in scanning equipment and facilities, but also ongoing technical support from various experts, including psychiatrists, physicists, neuroscientists, computer programmers, psychologists, and biostatisticians. The administrative costs of research have also risen in recent years because of increasing institutional and governmental oversight aimed at protecting the rights and safety of research participants and at ensuring that research dollars are well utilized (Holmes et al., 2000; Miller, 2001; Shalala, 2000).

The above discussion characterizes the challenges of obtaining funding for GME and research activity more generally. Most of these constraints are not unique to psychiatry, but affect other branches of medical practice and research as well. Constraints on these resource streams logically translate into a short supply of money to finance the research training activities of residents and the underlying infrastructure needed to support that training.

A Business Case for Research

Despite the above financial limitations, many programs incorporate research and research training into their broad departmental activities. They do so largely because new knowledge, especially as it relates to enhancing patient care, fits naturally into the philosophy of most clinical departments and institutions. Nevertheless, the ideal of research and research training can be at odds with the immediate needs of patients and the financial bottom line of departments. Accordingly, the committee believes a specific business case for research and research training should be aggressively pursued by psychiatry departments and should be formalized as part of a department's financial plan. This business case should include metrics to measure both the direct and indirect benefits of research activity and research training within a department.

Regarding the direct financial benefits of research, the committee was able to identify only one study, by Chin et al. (1985), that compares research-generated departmental income with income from clinical activity. This study found that research activities yielded far more departmental revenue per faculty FTE than the faculty clinical practice plan ($944,000/year versus $250,000/year).[25] Chin et al's. work is based on 1981 data from a large and relatively wealthy department (Stanford University's Department of Internal Medicine), so it has limited contemporary applicability and does not necessarily support a business case for research in less resource-intensive settings. Furthermore, Chin et al. do not factor in the resources necessary to support faculty during periods when grants are not funded or clinical volumes are not achieved. Never-

---

[25] Based on a sample of 52 FTEs who, on average, spent 27 percent of their time on federal or other extramurally funded research.

theless, the study does indicate that departments can develop measures of the financial return related to research activity.

Metrics or accounting systems have been developed to quantify the departmental income and relative value of research compared with other activities, including clinical and teaching responsibilities (Kastor et al., 1997; Scheid et al., 2002). Although the committee is not aware of any studies that have used metrics to demonstrate the financial benefits of a sustained research effort by medical departments, it is reasonable to hypothesize that such metrics could help individual departments determine the feasibility of using intramural resources to pursue the goal of building an extramurally funded research portfolio. Finally, analogous metrics could be used to assess less direct benefits of department-supported research, such as the prestige or faculty or patron satisfaction associated with research activity. Specifically, successful research programs are likely to attract the most ambitious faculty and trainees, as well as patients, third-party payers, and benefactors who are interested in having access to and supporting cutting-edge technologies (Pardes, 2002).

Strategies for Funding Smaller Programs

Building a research program or research training effort in less resource-intensive settings is more challenging than sustaining a large, existing program. The current reality is that some institutions receive considerable federal funding, whereas the rest receive little or none (Brainard, 2002). Psychiatry is no exception in this regard, as most psychiatric research funding is concentrated in the top 10 to 15 percent of psychiatry departments nationwide (Pincus, 2002). Specifically, in 2002 the top 10 NIH-funded departments obtained a combined total of nearly $365 million, while the next 75 departments received a total of $386 million (NIH, 2003b). For child and adolescent psychiatry, the concentration of research wealth is even greater, with fewer than 10 child and adolescent divisions having a substantial research effort (Beresin, 1997). In internal medicine departments, by comparison, the concentration of research resources is less severe, with the top 10 departments obtaining a total of $893 million, compared with $1.615 billion for the next 75 departments (NIH, 2003b). Thus the top 10 departments in psychiatry obtained nearly 49 percent of NIH funding for that discipline, whereas the top 10 in internal medicine received only 36 percent of the corresponding aggregate funding. Consequently, it may well be that many or most psychiatry departments lack the technological infrastructure and critical mass of researchers necessary to effectively support comprehensive research activity and training.

The obvious way for these smaller departments to build a research and research training effort is to seek extramural support. However, the disparity between resource-rich and resource-poor programs makes it difficult for the latter to compete for extramural support because funding agencies, especially those that fund training or early career award grants, are interested in the resources and environment of the applicants' institution, including the qualifications of mentors or senior investigators. The general challenge of obtaining extramural funding has become even greater because the NIH budget-doubling initiative is complete as of 2003, and because significant declines have occurred in the U.S. economy since early 2001.

Nevertheless, numerous private and public extramural funding options exist for biomedical researchers. Appendix B lists several government, foundation, and industry grants that support research training or research infrastructure during or in close temporal proximity to residency. Some of the sources of extramural research support are also summarized below.

Large grants from NIH. Building infrastructure is important to small programs that wish to compete with larger institutions, attract quality researchers, and sustain research efforts. Two infrastructure grants—the Centers of Biomedical Research Excellence (COBRE) and the Biomedical Research Infrastructure Network (BRIN)—target 23 states and Puerto Rico, as these localities have historically been low utilizers of NIH funding mechanisms. Accordingly, these mechanisms may be models for the establishment of research infrastructure at institutions with less resource-intensive departments of psychiatry.

The BRIN and COBRE grants are designed to build local biomedical research infrastructure, including personnel recruitment and training efforts, in regions having the greatest need for resource expansion. Considering that more than 50 percent of all NIMH funding goes to four states (New York, California, Pennsylvania, and Massachusetts)[26] (NIMH, 2001a), it appears reasonable for departments of psychiatry in other states to consider these infrastructure-building grant mechanisms or other funding opportunities that target underrepresented regions or small departments. NIMH might encourage applications for these or similar funding mechanisms by marketing them more aggressively to small or emerg-

---

[26] Census data for 2000 indicate that the population in these four states is 27 percent of the entire U.S. population.

ing programs, and by encouraging resource-rich programs to partner with smaller programs such that the latter can enhance their research efforts while the former work to expand their geographic perspective and access to patient populations.

The first BRIN (3 years in duration) and COBRE (5 years in duration) grants were awarded in 2000 and 2001, respectively. The BRIN grant is aimed at fostering collaboration among different institutions within one state, whereas the COBRE grant is awarded to one institution that may or may not collaborate with others. The BRIN grant encourages the creation of a research infrastructure that will attract research scientists. The COBRE grant operates with one senior scientist who fosters the development of junior investigators; to receive a COBRE grant, an institution must establish three to five multidisciplinary research projects. The maximum amount given to a state for a BRIN grant is $2 million/year (each state may submit no more than two applications for potential funding) (NIH, 2000b). The maximum amount given to an institution for a COBRE grant is $1.5 million/year, with a limit of three simultaneous submissions (NIH, 2001b; 2002c).

As of spring 2003, most research projects funded under these infrastructure mechanisms support basic research, although clinical research is permitted. None of the funded grants focus on training psychiatry residents, although approximately 40 percent have a neuroscience component. The projects funded thus far are reviewed individually on an annual basis. A systematic and broad review of their overall success in terms of research productivity is not anticipated until 2004 (personal communication, F. Taylor, National Center for Research Resources, April 10, 2003).

The NIH General Clinical Research Center (GCRC) grant is another model that can be used by NIH and other institutions to build research programs at less research-intensive institutions. Departments should consider these centers for the development of fledging research projects and training opportunities. Approximately 80 GCRCs currently support inpatient and outpatient facilities, core laboratories, bioinformatics programs, biostatisticians, and administrative technical personnel, all of which can be utilized by subscribing investigators at relatively modest cost (AAMC, 1999). Several GCRCs across the country have behavioral assessment cores that can assist with psychiatric research efforts (NIH, 2003a). Although these centers are at large, well-established institutions and are intended to support established investigators with peer-reviewed research funding, NIH encourages GCRCs to expand their efforts by supporting new training and research grants. Specifically, this means GCRCs are encouraged to support fledgling investigators conducting pilot studies and ultimately aiming to submit training or other grant applications themselves. GCRCs can support these new investigators or trainees by offering logistic (e.g., human subject informed consent), scientific (e.g., statistical), and infrastructure (e.g., inpatient and outpatient facilities) resources.

Industry or philanthropic support. There are numerous other sources of research and research training funds in addition to the federal funding mechanisms described above and in Appendix B. In a presentation to the committee in June 2002, Herbert Pardes, chief executive officer (CEO), New York Presbyterian Hospital (former director of NIMH), suggested that surplus income from industry-sponsored trials could be earmarked for departmental research. Dependence on industry funding, however, has drawbacks, as the work can be tedious and also can involve conflicts of interest (IOM, 1994; 2002b; Pincus, 1995). Therefore, such arrangements with industry need to be carefully conceived.

Dr. Pardes and others have also made the point that medical institutions need to work aggressively to raise money for research from private sources, such as foundations and individuals in their community (Jacobs et al., 1997; Pardes, 2002). This notion is supported by public opinion surveys indicating that 61 percent of the population is willing to pay higher taxes to support research funding (Research!America, 2002), as well as by focus group and survey work done by the AAMC revealing that biomedical research and patient care rank well ahead of clinical GME in the minds of most voting Americans (Knapp, 2002). These findings indicate that general departmental fund-raising efforts and those targeting residency or fellowship research training programs are of interest to many potential private donors. In fact, philanthropic support for GME might well benefit from reminding potential donors that today's residents are tomorrow's researchers. One example of successful philanthropic fund raising occurred at the University of Texas at Southwestern, where the psychiatry department raised funds to support nine endowed chairs, four additional faculty positions, and $18 million in research activities from 1977 to 1996 (Meyer and McLaughlin, 1998).

Collaboration with other departments or institutions. An alternative way for small programs to tap available clinical research resources is to seek out opportunities for interdepartmental or interinstitutional collaboration. A recent AAMC task force made the following recommendation:

> To enhance clinical research programs and infrastructure development, medical schools and teaching hospitals

should encourage interdepartmental collaborations, as well as joint efforts and alliances with other units in the university and with external organizations, such as community organizations, HMOs, and other medical schools and teaching hospitals (AAMC, 1999:80).

In a 1998 study of how psychiatry is adapting to the pressures of managed care, Meyer and McLaughlin (1998:84) also advocate a broad collaborative approach:

As individual clinical departments become less able to fund their own essential research infrastructure, medical schools will need to develop institution-wide collaborative efforts to assure access to cutting-edge technology relevant to research on clinical disorders. In this regard, research in psychiatry may be linked to other efforts in clinical and basic neuroscience, human genetics, health services research, clinical trials, and treatment and prevention research relative to general and mental health issues.

Meyer and McLaughlin cite several examples of successful collaborations between researchers lacking critical technology and those having the necessary resources. One such example is Meyer's experience as chair at the University of Connecticut's department of psychiatry, during which time an addiction "center without walls" was formed between his program and Yale University's Department of Psychiatry. Since the center's formation, principal investigators have come from both the Yale and University of Connecticut faculty (Meyer and McLaughlin, 1998). The University of Connecticut's current program is described further in the section below on curriculum.

LEADERSHIP AND MENTORING

Institutional Leadership

It is perhaps axiomatic to say that if research endeavors are important to presidents of universities, CEOs of hospitals, and deans of medical schools, research will be important to department heads, training directors, and residents. Many of those who made presentations to the committee—including Herbert Pardes; Paula Clayton, former chair, department of psychiatry, University of Minnesota; and Henry Nasrallah, former chair, department of psychiatry, Ohio State University—made this point (Clayton, 2002; Nasrallah, 2002; Pardes, 2002). Additionally, the literature contains numerous references to the importance of leadership to the research endeavor, psychiatric research, and research training (Katerndahl, 1996; Meyer and McLaughlin, 1998; Pardes and Pincus, 1983; Rosenberg, 1999).

Leaders who value research will likely promote research and research training in the following ways:

- They will recruit department and division heads who have research experience.
- They will consider research a major part of their leadership agenda, thereby advancing institutional comprehension of the value of research activity.
- They will use research success as an important criterion for appointment and promotion, taking into consideration the challenges associated with patient-oriented research.
- They are more likely to offer research start-up funds and other resources to newly hired faculty so these individuals will have time to prepare competitive applications for extramural funding.
- They will offer qualified faculty provisions for unfunded release time from other activities (e.g., clinical and administrative) for purposes of initiating or renewing extramural research funding streams. These release time provisions may furthermore be offered to offset the time necessary to teach and mentor trainees and medical students.
- They will encourage trainees to engage in ongoing or original research projects, and raise and distribute money for capital enhancements to the research infrastructure, including space, equipment, and administrative support personnel (AAMC, 2002b; Ahrens, 1992; Kaplan, 2000).

These executive strategies for research promotion are perhaps obvious, and there is evidence that many leaders in academic medicine appreciate and support the importance of the research enterprise, including clinical research. However, there is also concern that many leaders say they support research on the one hand, but overemphasize the financial bottom line in favor of clinical revenues on the other (Oinonen et al., 2001; Rosenberg, 1999).

Departmental Leadership

In addition to support from institutional executives, the department chair's attitude is critical to fostering research and research training. According to Paula Clayton in her presentation to the committee (2002), the chair has principal authority over professional expectations that include the amount of time devoted by faculty and residents to various activities, including research. To advance the goal of increasing patient-oriented psychiatrist-researchers, the committee believes it is best if department chairs are themselves successful basic or patient-oriented researchers. In lieu of that direct experience, the chair might designate an associate chair who is an accomplished researcher. Having a researcher in a leadership role gives investigative efforts the necessary voice to request department resources and to characterize the importance of emerging knowledge to trainees as well as to the general public.

Although based largely on presentations to the committee by chairs and resident training directors of psychiatry departments, our strong view is that when hospital executives and department chairs view research as a high priority, there is an increased likelihood that research and research training programs—including research-focused didactics, biostatistical and data management support, research options for residents, department-sponsored research fellowships, effective mentorship, and funding for travel to attend national research meetings—will flourish. Empirical support for the importance of leadership is difficult to obtain, but at least one recent study offers validation of the notion that proactive leadership can promote research activity. A study of 351 departments of family medicine (76 percent response rate) found that research activity, quantified by the number of publications and funded grants, increased in large programs (i.e., those with more than nine faculty) that had a strategic research plan and in small programs (i.e., those with nine or fewer faculty) that mandated research activity among faculty members. Comparable increases were not seen in those that did not have such research mandates (Kruse et al., 2003).

In accordance with requirements established by the Psychiatry Residency Review Committee (RRC), accredited training programs must have a residency program director who devotes at least half-time effort to the administration of the residency program (ACGME, 2000b). Training directors typically remain in their position for a very short time: 30 percent vacate their position each year, and most occupy the position for less than 3 years (Balon and Singh, 2001; Batalden et al., 2002; Miller, 2002; Winstead, 2001). Research experience is neither a prequalification nor a common characteristic of the vast majority of training directors

(ACGME, 2000b; Dawkins, 2002; Drell, 2002). Given that training directors interact with residents more than do other department faculty, the committee believes the ideal research training program in residency will have an experienced researcher as the training director, although we acknowledge that there may not be enough psychiatrist-researchers to fill that role (Drell, 2002). Alternatively, and in line with the time demands of the program directorship, a researcher can be appointed, perhaps as an associate, to participate in structuring an educational program for residents that will include exposure to practical and theoretical research opportunities. Regardless of exactly how researchers are better integrated into the departmental education effort, encouragement from senior leadership will likely be of critical importance to a program's ultimate ability to secure resources and motivate trainees to pursue research education and careers.

Mentorship

Mentorship is arguably the most intense and critical form of leadership associated with training in any field. It is one of the most frequently cited components of a successful biomedical research career (Balon and Singh, 2001; Blake et al., 1994; DeHaven et al., 1998; IOM, 1994; Kanigel, 1993; Ledley and Lovejoy, 1993; Lewinsohn et al., 1998; National Research Council [NRC], 1997; Pincus et al., 1995). An IOM report on careers in clinical research notes:

> Mentors play a crucial role in stimulating individuals to pursue a particular career path, shaping the content of their training, socializing them in the research environment, and providing support and guidance in the formative stages of their career (IOM, 1994:58).

Several surveys of M.D.-researchers have led to the conclusion that mentoring is one of the most important influences on career choice for potential physician-investigators (Balon and Singh, 2001; DeHaven et al., 1998; Levey, 1992; Levey et al., 1988; Pincus et al., 1995; Shapiro et al., 1991). A survey by Pincus et al. (1995), for example, found that more than 95 percent of respondents cited time with a mentor as an extremely important part of their research training, more important than other training components assessed. And a survey of 20 psychiatry residency training directors found that "the one point on which there was general agreement was that the most important way of interesting a resident in research is to provide successful experience with a research mentor" (Rieder, 1988:288).

Several participants at the committee's workshop on obstacles to research training (see Appendix A) spoke of the importance of mentors and the scarcity of time for researchers to serve in that role. Martin Drell of Louisiana State University (former president of the American Association of Directors of Psychiatry Residency Training [AADPRT]) said that residents look to their training directors and clinical supervisors, who are nonresearchers, for inspiration. Furthermore, he added that researchers typically do not spend time with medical students or residents:

> If you are truly serious about being a researcher, you eschew everything else, such as teaching, to become totally focused on your research career....As you get more successful in research, you remove yourself more from the very population that could probably benefit from your inspiration.

At the committee's September 2002 meeting, Daniel Winstead, chair, department of psychiatry and neurology, Tulane University (recent chair of the Psychiatry RRC, current member of the board of directors of the American Board of Psychiatry and Neurology, and president of the American Association of Chairs of Departments of Psychiatry), was even stronger in his assessment of the lack of interaction between researchers and nonresearchers in psychiatry. He suggested that researchers and nonresearchers in psychiatry exist in "different worlds" that include different organizations, meetings, committees, and faculty tracks (Winstead, 2002). As psychiatrists in their formative years tend to gravitate toward one world or the other, and as there are few patient-oriented researchers in psychiatry, these professional differences limit opportunities for potential researchers to meet and pair with suitable mentors.

In his presentation to the committee, Roger Meyer, a psychiatrist and senior consultant for clinical research at the AAMC, summarized the situation as follows: "Most medical students and residents are not being systematically exposed to high-quality clinical research or role models and mentors as part of their professional development" (Meyer, 2002).

The current lack of psychiatrists in the academic community who specialize in child and adolescent psychiatry makes the shortage of suitable mentors for residents in that subspecialty especially acute. According to a study by the AADPRT, child and adolescent programs are small

(75 percent have six or fewer faculty), and nearly half of those programs have problems recruiting high-quality faculty (Beresin, 1997; Beresin and Borus, 1989). Special efforts must be made to address mentorship in child and adolescent psychiatry programs. Moreover, given the shortage of child and adolescent psychiatrists serving as research mentors, departments should develop mentoring arrangements between child and adolescent trainees and faculty in other divisions and departments.

Recognizing the importance of mentoring early in a resident's training, the Western Psychiatric Institute and Clinic's (WPIC) department of psychiatry provides a network of mentors to residents early in their training. By providing more than a single mentor to each trainee, this system increases the probability that suitable mentor matching will occur during the residency period. For example, some faculty may mentor students on how to find a suitable mentor or project, whereas others may ultimately offer the trainee an individualized research education (Pincus, 2001a; 2002; Swartz and Cho, 2002). While such multitiered mentoring requires additional faculty and is potentially redundant, the committee believes it represents a wise approach given the complex interpersonal and scientific issues than can underlie the formation and maintenance of the mentor–trainee relationship (Kanigel, 1993).

At present, psychiatry appears to be open to broad sources of mentoring, including joint mentoring by junior and senior faculty and the use of visiting or even remote professors as mentors (Lewinsohn et al., 1998). Psychiatrists also depend heavily on Ph.D. mentors, as psychologists (including many clinical psychologists) and other non-M.D. doctorates represent nearly 60 percent of NIH-funded investigators in departments of psychiatry (Meyer, 2002).[27] Indeed, the shortage of mentor time is considered so acute that for smaller programs, remote or telementoring might be an effective remedy. An example of how such remote mentoring can be accomplished is provided by the Service Corps of Retired Executives (SCORE), a nonprofit association of 11,500 volunteer business counselors. The association provides e-mail counseling to "aspiring entrepreneurs" and especially targets small-business owners (SCORE, 2003). The American Psychiatric Association colloquium (APA, 2003), the minority mentoring network (National Advisory Mental Health Council's Workgroup on Racial/Ethnic Diversity in Research Training and Health Disparities Research, 2001), and a summer seminar series in geriatrics (Halpain et al., 2001) are three programs in psychiatry that

---

[27] In 1999, 59 percent of NIH grant awardees in departments of psychiatry held a Ph.D. degree. By comparison, Ph.D.'s in internal medicine departments hold 24 percent of that discipline's NIH grants.

could form the foundation for a SCORE-like mentoring network or some other national project to connect trainees to mentors. Although remote mentoring would likely prove to be far inferior to in-person training, it might nevertheless foster collaborations between senior and fledgling investigators that would otherwise not occur. It might also ignite research careers among some talented trainees.

Despite the widely acknowledged importance of good mentoring, there are strong financial and time obstacles to faculty members' mentoring of residents, fellows, and junior colleagues. Medical school faculty members are expected to account for their time in generating the bulk of the funding for their salaries. Most faculty costs associated with research training and mentoring must be subsidized either by the sponsoring institution or by the faculty member's taking time from other funded activities. The latter strategy is problematic given increased scrutiny and accountability for the allocation of federal resources. In addition, as a result of increased clinical loads, lower clinical revenues, and/or the general demands of research, many academic clinicians have difficulty finding the time to mentor. As noted by the AAMC Task Force on Clinical Research (1999:63), reduced time for mentoring is coupled with lower revenues from clinical work:

> Faculty practice and affiliated hospital revenues have been major sources of discretionary funds for the subsidy of research....As pressures have mounted to sustain clinical income on lower rates of reimbursement per patient, faculty in these departments have difficulty accessing time for research and research mentorship.

For those departments with solid funding and a supply of talented trainees, trainees serve as much-valued junior colleagues. For smaller programs and those with a limited supply of trainees or resources, training a new researcher may initially require a considerable expenditure of time with little gain. It has been suggested by some established researchers that one way to counter the lack of funding for mentors is to provide supplemental funding to senior investigators who commit time to mentoring young investigators (Lewinsohn et al., 1998; Meador-Woodruff, 2002). Such piecewise funding may be especially relevant to research progress at institutions with limited resources and to trainees who have little or no research experience. There is at least one grant mechanism—the federally funded Midcareer Investigator Award in Patient-oriented Research (or K24 grant)—that explicitly funds established investigators to develop their skills as clinical researchers *and* as mentors. This award, which has a duration of up to 5 years, allows clinical researchers 50 percent time to develop these skills. NIH funds 60 to 80 K24 awards each year (NIH, 1999c). In general, however, salary support under research and training grants does not include mentor salaries because of the philosophy that (1) teaching is compensated by the productivity of the trainee, and (2) teaching is part of the core responsibilities of an academician and of their sponsoring institution. Given the shortage of mentors and the fact that many mentors have time constraints secondary to increased service requirements, it appears logical to the committee that a broader array of support mechanisms is needed to make mentoring a more frequent part of residency training.

PROGRAM AND CURRICULUM STRUCTURE

Central to a program's ability to train researchers are the structure of the departmental milieu and the training curriculum. This section explores those elements in four ways. First, it reviews existing literature that describes various clinical training programs both within and outside of psychiatry. Second, it describes five illustrative training models, drawing on a combination of the published literature and communications between the committee and program faculty. Third, it presents the views of eight department chairs whose programs the committee believes can be characterized as emerging with regard to their overall research effort and exemplify various strategies and ideas for enhancing research training options in residency training. Finally, it details informal information gathered from several child and adolescent psychiatry divisions that characterizes the issues they face regarding research.

Published Reports on Research Curriculum Design

A number of publications address clinical research training both within and outside of psychiatry, but only a small number of these reports focus on residency; even fewer consider program success by offering substantive outcome data (i.e., information about how effective the program has actually been at training productive researchers). The absence of solid literature on research training in residency is likely related to the reality that medical educators are typically trained as medical doctors, and focus first on content rather than on established educational methods (Sheets and Anderson, 1991). Nevertheless, there are some worthwhile publications addressing research training in clinical research broadly and in psychiatry more specifically. Some of these works are reviewed below. It should be noted that these publications represent an illustrative sampling rather than a systematic review of all existing literature on the subject. This sampling emphasizes clinical research training for all M.D.'s generally, and especially for potential psychiatrists. All the works reviewed are from the last 10 years.

An excellent summary of existing training programs was produced by the AAMC Task Force on Clinical Research (1999). This summary describes 16 illustrative programs to demonstrate the range of contexts and issues that relate to clinical research training. A majority of programs lead to masters or Ph.D. degrees, although a small number are short-term (e.g., summer programs). The fact that these programs are so variable in length led the task force to conclude that the optimal length for clinical training is unclear. All programs place a high value on intensive, hands-on training in conjunction with requisite coursework. Common core training courses include biostatistics, epidemiology, grant writing, and design and methodology of clinical trials. Mentored research is noted as a key component of these programs. Funding for salaries (of trainees and mentors), tuition, and administrative costs are key constraints on program size and effectiveness. Trainee recruitment at most institutions is not considered a major problem. Instead, "converting...[potential trainee] interest into a solid career choice" is viewed as a greater challenge. Finally, these descriptions do not identify programs that integrate research training into conventional residency, although they encompass options that couple subspecialty training with a Ph.D. in clinical investigation (e.g., The Johns Hopkins University's Graduate Training Program in Clinical Investigation), a part-time masters degrees, or "time out" from residency options.

An important model described by the AAMC task force is the NIH Clinical Research Curriculum Development Award (or K30 grant) developed in response to a 1997 NIH report on clinical research (known as the Nathan Report). This grant offers support for the creation of clinical research training curricula for postdoctoral-level trainees across disciplines (NIH, 1997b). Wide latitude is given to the institution to develop a curriculum that suits its local needs, but a typical implementation resembles a 2-year masters degree. As the program is new, no evaluation has yet been done, and it is not clear how long the program will continue (personal communication, L. Friedman, NIH, April 17, 2003). Nevertheless, the K30 is relevant to residency-based research training because it encourages the development of clear educational goals related to general clinical research training. As of April 2003, an informal e-mail posting to 57 K30 program directors had yielded a response from 21 programs, reporting a total of 556 trainees. Those programs all indicated that they were designed to accommodate full-time fellows and junior faculty; thus, only 2 percent of the trainees were residents, and 1 percent were psychiatrists. Low resident utilization of existing K30 grants suggests that psychiatry departments need to increase their trainees' awareness of the K30 program at their institution. It may further suggest that few if any implemented K30 programs have been designed to accommodate the intense schedules to which residents must adhere.

A systematic literature review by Hebert et al. (2003) identifies 41 publications focused specifically on residency-based research training among different specialties. The search criteria included only published curricula describing local programs that target research training for residents. Hebert et al. found only a single program designed to produce academic physicians, suggesting that most programs are directing their research training efforts to all residents rather than to the training of independent physician-investigators. The authors further note that evaluation procedures are used infrequently: only 12 percent of the publications include some objective measures of pre- and postintervention research skills or accomplishments, and none include long-term follow-up.

The obvious conclusion one can draw from Hebert et al.'s review is that, somewhat ironically, literature on research training is not very scientific. It does, however, provide anecdotes and knowledgeable opinions regarding frequently endorsed goals and obstacles to research training. Given the earlier discussion in this chapter, it is not surprising that lack of time and money are key barriers noted explicitly in 7 of the 41 publications. Additionally, with regard to mentoring, 6 articles cite lack of faculty experience in supervising residents in research as a barrier. Somewhat surprising is the fact that resistance from residents is identified as an obstacle to research training in 8 articles. Key goals cited most frequently are attaining competency in critical review of research findings (13 articles) and increasing the actual scholarly activity of residents (14 articles).

In January 2000, Balon and Singh surveyed 126 academic departments of psychiatry in North America with a brief (30-item) questionnaire aimed at research training (2001). The survey yielded a modest response rate of 59 percent, in part because the subject matter likely elicited a higher proportional response rate from research-intensive training programs than from more clinically oriented programs. Aggregated findings include the following percentages that summarize the status of research training in psychiatry. Of the 70 responses received, just under a third of the programs have a research track, and for 87 percent of those programs, fewer than one in four residents enter that track. A high proportion (91 percent) of all programs have a research elective month, which is typically offered in PGY3 or PGY4 (78 percent of the time). Fewer than half of the programs (42 percent) offer a research fellowship. Nearly all the programs (91 percent) offer a research course to residents, most typically in PGY2 (48 percent). This research coursework usually accounts for less than 6 percent of the entire curriculum. Courses in research design are rarely part of the didactic (28 percent), and although most programs provide the "opportunity" for residents to join a research project, in 73 percent of the programs, fewer than 25 percent of the residents actually do so. Overall, the survey led the authors to conclude that research didactic learning and activity in academic psychiatry departments of North America are insufficient.

Several recent articles review local efforts to increase research training among residents. Clayton and Sheldon-Keller (2001) describe a weekly 1-hour mandatory seminar for PGY2 residents that involved group engineering, implementation, and research/writing of a modest research project. Between 1994 and 2001, 30 residents took part in the seminar. Satisfaction ratings were favorable, although not outstanding, and simple pre- and post-testing of 13 to 14 residents indicated that they had gained research knowledge from the experience. The authors note the value of linking short-term activities to the formal process of conveying scientific results to the outside community of scientists (e.g., literature searches and reviews are conceptually linked to the production of manuscript or grant "background" sections).

Paniagua et al. (1993) describe a weekly 2-hour research seminar, during which child and adolescent psychiatry residents reviewed case vignette modules that included a list of pertinent research questions. The philosophy behind this training was to emphasize the relevance of research to the future development of psychiatric practice. Of the 14 trainees who participated in the program from 1989 to 1991, 8 developed research projects, and 5 became academicians (Paniagua et al., 1993). Paniagua et al. also emphasize the importance of translating research material into a language that is readily comprehensible to individuals with clinical medical training.

Lambert and Garver (1998) describe a program for mentoring of medical students and psychiatric residents in publishing a scientific paper. They suggest that such a program is of central importance to effective research training based on the premise that publishing a paper is "one of the most rewarding experiences in academic life..." (Lambert and Garver, 1998:47). They also stated that the program was implemented in 1992 despite skepticism by many faculty who "had reservations about investing large amounts of time and energy if most residents were unenthusiastic about the endeavor" (Lambert and Garver, 1998:48). As an index of the program's success they report that by 1995 eight papers were produced by an equal number of residents. These papers ranged from case reports by junior faculty to a formal empirical study by a fourth-year resident on a 9-month research track.

Pato and Pato (2001), former faculty at the State University of New York at Buffalo (currently at the State University of New York at Syracuse), describe a seminar consisting of 12 1-hour lectures designed to teach psychiatry residents the process of research. The first 8 lectures were aimed at various types of study designs (e.g., case-control); the last 4 focused on research writing and publishing. At the end of the seminar, all participants submitted a "letter to the editor." Outcome data using pre- and postseminar measures to assess subjective (i.e., self-assessment) and objective gains in research knowledge were favorable, although the practical impact of the work product was more limited: of 74 participants in the seminar, 68 had submitted letters to the editor, but only 13 of those letters had been published (Pato and Pato, 2001). More important, no data are presented about the career paths since taken by the seminar participants. Nevertheless, this intervention is notable for its portability, as it is adaptable to various topics in psychiatric research, and the authors themselves have implemented the program in at least two other institutions besides their own.

Kirchner et al. (1998) describe a departmental effort to increase research activity among residents at the University of Arkansas for Medical Sciences. The system utilized a block rotation through multiple affiliated training sites, including the Central Arkansas Veterans Healthcare System, the state psychiatric hospital, and affiliated outpatient clinics. Most of the sites offered residents the opportunity to join ongoing research activities. These arrangements included a research training option that provided at least 1 half-day of protected research time and 1 hour of supervision per week. The department also established a standing committee of faculty representatives, including the residency training director, to oversee residency-based research activities and to review residents and faculty involved in these research training arrangements. Other general features of the program included a formal assessment of PGY1 residents' knowledge and interests regarding research, and PGY3 and PGY4 rotations in an outpatient clinic that included an ongoing research effort in depression treatment outcomes. As an index of the success of the overall program, the authors note that resident-authored abstracts and resident research activity have since increased. More specific or long-term assessment of participants is not reported.

A number of common themes emerge from the above literature review. First, the timing and duration of clinical research training are quite variable. Some programs offer Ph.D. degrees, others masters, and others only an isolated experience with no formal certificate. Generically, clinical research programs offer instruction in biostatistics, epidemiology, paper and grant writing, clinical trials design, and research study critiquing skills. Research training across medical residencies is limited by time and the desires of many residents who presumably are focused on completing their clinical training. Nevertheless, many programs are striving to increase scholarly activity among their residents. Research training exists within psychiatric residency, but intensive research training in the form of research tracks appears to attract fewer than 9 percent of residents (Balon and Singh, 2001). For the successful programs that do exist, only limited data are available on the long-term effectiveness of their efforts (i.e., the career research productivity of their trainees).

Illustrative Programs

This section describes five illustrative programs that appear to have amassed exceptional research-related resources. The programs of Columbia University, WPIC, and the University of Michigan are included because they have been recognized as illustrative research training programs by NIMH and APA. The committee wishes to note that a description of the University of Michigan's program is retained despite the fact that one of the committee members is from that program. Michigan's program, however, is described because it offers a useful example of how intermediate-sized programs can foster research training efforts. The University of Connecticut's program was also selected because it represents an intermediate-sized program with a developing research training effort. Finally, the NIMH PGY4 program is highlighted because of its connection to the world-class biomedical research environment of NIH. As noted earlier, these five programs should be considered a sample of convenience, used by the committee to detail the current state of research training by highlighting those programs that, at least by reputation, appear to be succeeding in their research effort generally and by extension at research training. These five programs should not be taken as an exhaustive list of high-quality or up-and-coming research training programs in psychiatry, as there clearly are other successful programs not described here, including those closely affiliated with the committee members authoring this report.

Columbia University

One of the largest psychiatric residency research training programs is that of the New York Presbyterian Hospital and the New York State Psychiatric Institute (NYSPI). The program is administered by Columbia University's department of psychiatry, a department that is closely coupled with numerous research efforts at Columbia and the NYSPI. These research efforts include a neurobiology division directed by Nobel laureate Eric Kandel and the Center for Psychoanalytic Training and Research, established in 1945, the first such alliance between psychoanalysts and a university in the United States. The program's curriculum and overall environment are detailed on the department's website (Columbia University, 2002), and its research training philosophy was recently featured in an issue of the APA's *Psychiatric Research Report* (Rieder, 2003).

The core didactic curriculum includes approximately 525 hours of instruction distributed across PGY2 through PGY4 (Columbia University, 2002). The didactics are dominated by clinical training. Only in PGY4 is there formal instruction in psychiatric research and in "journal reading," amounting jointly to 13 hours of classroom time. The strong implication of such a curriculum is twofold. First, psychiatric educators at Columbia University believe that the mastery of clinical knowledge, ranging from psychopharmacology to psychotherapy, should dominate the early core didactic curriculum of the psychiatry residency. Second, researchers who emerge from Columbia's residency program do so in large part because of longitudinal experiences that occur outside of the didactic curriculum. The residency program, for instance, places some PGY1 residents in the schizophrenia research unit for 3 months and all PGY2 residents in a research unit for nonpsychotic disorders for 4 months. Residents also have opportunities for research work with a "preceptor" during PGY2 and PGY3 and up to 8 months of elective research in PGY4. Finally, all residents are required to conduct an independent study project that may include preparing a research paper for publication (Columbia University, 2002).

These residency program components suggest an implicit research track for at least some residents, although it is notable that Columbia recently discontinued its formal research track in favor of encouraging all residents to pursue research experiences (personal communication, R. Rieder, Columbia University, March 29, 2003). Ultimately, however, Columbia's residency training aims to educate the next generation of psychiatrist-researchers by encouraging residents to extend their training to a 2- to 4-year research fellowship. These fellowships, mentioned previously, offer intense training in nine different topic areas (e.g., substance abuse, schizophrenia, child psychiatry), and stipends are supported with training funds from NIMH (T32) and the state. Data for 1989 to 1998 suggest that 60 to 70 percent of fellowship graduates in schizophrenia and affective disorders maintained careers as researchers by obtaining either an early mentored career (K) award (45 percent) or other full-time support for their academic efforts (24 percent) (Rieder, 2003). It is also notable that female and minority graduates from these fellowships have been successful in sustaining research careers at rates comparable to those for men and nonminorities (Rieder, 2003). For residents, however, research career tracking is less common, as only 56 of 184 graduates (or 30 percent) from 1985 to 1999 moved on to research careers (personal communication, R. Rieder, Columbia University, April 10, 2003).

Western Psychiatric Institute and Clinic

WPIC in Pittsburgh is the leading psychiatry department in terms of total funding received from NIH. In fiscal year 2002, it received nearly $78 million in federal funding (NIH, 2003b). As is the case with the Columbia residency, most lecture and seminar time is devoted to clinical issues, although there is an "advanced literature seminar" in PGY3 (WPIC, 2002a). The implication once again is that dedicated research training courses are not typical, even in a research-intensive program. Yet while research is not necessarily central to lectures and seminars, residents at WPIC likely obtain research exposure because of the research culture that exists at the institution. The department chair is David Kupfer, and his commitment to psychiatric research and research training is well established (Kupfer et al., 2002; Meyer and McLaughlin, 1998). Indeed, the values of departmental leadership have been noted as supremely relevant to the institution's successes in overall research activity (Pincus, 2002). Mentoring, also said to be key to WPIC's success, is made possible by the "critical mass" of researchers: the department has more than 100 faculty principal investigators (WPIC, 2002c). There is also an incentive for mentoring in that success in the activity is a significant criterion for promotion (Swartz and Cho, 2002). The importance of the interpersonal aspects of research training is further emphasized by monthly dinner meetings of trainees and senior faculty that typically occur at the vice chair's home.

As noted earlier, trainee research activity at WPIC has been linked conceptually to research training experiences before and after residency (see Table 2-1 in Chapter 2). This linkage is characterized as a "series of bridges" that help psychiatric trainees deal with the path from medical school to independent investigator status (Swartz and Cho, 2002). As with the program at Columbia, several T32 fellowships are available at WPIC. Additionally, there is an R25 grant (see Appendix B for a brief description) that supports junior faculty time for grant preparation, as well as seminars in research survival skills targeting residents, fellows, and junior faculty. Entry into the research track in residency is informal, and about 50 percent of the residents who enter the research track do so at the beginning of their residency with others joining the track later during their training. Because of the clinical responsibilities in PGY1 and PGY2, research-related activities are held until the last 2 years of the adult residency and can involve as much as 50 percent time in PGY3 and nearly full time in PGY4. Outcome data indicate that from 1996 to 2001, at least 14 of 68 (21 percent) of graduating residents became research fellows (personal communication, N. Ryan, WPIC, April 16, 2003), and 11 of 17 R25 trainees from 1999 to 2002 received career awards (Swartz and Cho, 2002).

University of Michigan

Somewhat smaller than the programs at Columbia and WPIC is that at the University of Michigan. While Columbia and WPIC took in a combined $97.5 million in federal grant funds in 2002, the University of Michigan took in $9.6 million (NIH, 2003b). Nevertheless, Michigan's program is one of the models to which the psychiatric community has turned in the past few years in considering ways to enhance the integration of research training into the psychiatric residency. The Psychiatry Department at Michigan is well connected to efforts to enhance psychiatric research, as the chair of that department, John Greden, is also chair of the APA's Council on Research (see Chapter 3 for more detail).

The University of Michigan's model for research training in residency extends the 4-year adult psychiatric residency to 5 years so that the last 3 years of that training can include approximately 50 percent time for research activity (McCullum-Smith, 2002). This program was recently funded by an NIMH Mental Health Education Grant (R25) to cover the costs that are not encompassed by Medicare funding for residency training (NIH, 1999a). The program includes one or two 1-month research blocks in PGY2 to give residents some protected time to initiate their research projects. According to the vice chair for research at the University of Michigan, James Meador-Woodruff, as of November 2001, 90 percent of all graduates of this research track had moved on to research careers (Meador-Woodruff, 2001). Additional outcome data have not been obtained.

University of Connecticut

The program of the University of Connecticut's department of psychiatry, like that of the University of Michigan, is relatively small. The department received $4.6 million in NIH research funding in 2002, ranking forty-first among departments with regard to such extramural funding (NIH, 2003b). The department includes three prominent research centers: the Alcohol Research Center; the Neuropsychopharmacology Treatment, Research, and Training Center; and the Center for the Study of High Utilizers of Health Care. From 1997 to 2001, extramural research funding to the department increased from $7 million to $10 million, with most of that funding coming from the federal government and most being directed toward patient-oriented research.[28] The number of physician faculty members conducting research increased from 5 in 1997 to 12 in 2002. Within the entire 31-member department faculty, there have been 16 R01's and several career awards, one of which is described below.

Residents may pursue training in the 4-year adult residency program, subspecialty training in the 5-year child and adolescent psychiatry program, and/or a 1-year fellowship in clinical addiction psychiatry (begun in 1999 with funding from the National Institute on Alcohol Abuse and Alcoholism [NIAAA]) or a 2-year fellowship in psychopharmacology (begun in 2000) (University of Connecticut, 2002). Residents and other clinical investigators may also receive training in treatment outcomes for adolescents with alcohol or substance abuse problems under the supervision of Yifrah Kaminer, M.D., who received a K24 grant in 2002 from NIAAA. Those selected for this training program are provided general guidance and encouragement and are taught research methodology and data analysis (NIH, 1999a; University of Connecticut, 2002).

There are a number of seminars in each postgraduate year from which residents may choose, including several that focus on research methodology, clinical trials, informed consent, and ethics. Approximately 15 percent of the seminars offered deal with research and research-related issues. Additionally, PGY1 residents are rotated individually through a 1-month exploration of department research activities with no clinical obligations. Finally, a research requirement was initiated in 2001 whereby PGY1 residents attend a "research fair" that showcases departmental research, select a faculty mentor, conduct research during PGY2 through PGY4, and present findings during the Annual Research

---

[28] Unless otherwise indicated, data in this section were obtained through extensive personal communication with the department chair, Dr. Leighton Y. Huey.

Day. These programs appear to be steering more medical students and psychiatric residents toward patient-oriented research.

National Institute of Mental Health PGY4 Program

A survey of residency-based research training would be incomplete without including a program that is administered intramurally by NIMH, given that this program should have the best resources and students (NIMH, 2002b; 2002c). NIMH PGY4 program residents assume responsibility for the evaluation and clinical care of inpatient and/or outpatient research subjects at the state-of-the-art Warren Grant Magnuson Clinical Center. They also receive training in clinical research design, methodology, statistical analysis, and administration (e.g., funding, monitoring). In 2002, six adult and two child and adolescent psychiatry residents participated in the program. The program targets the most talented psychiatric residents in the country and aims to give them specialized training in biological psychiatric clinical research. It is not known how successful graduates of this program are at future research endeavors, as the program does not systematically follow the participants after graduation (personal communication, B. Kaplan, NIH, July 29, 2002).

Common Themes

One important theme that can be extracted from the above program descriptions is that there is typically a modest amount of research training in PGY1 and PGY2, with the exception of clinical rotations in research units (if they exist) and research-oriented didactics, which are likely to represent well under 10 percent of the resident's time. Some programs have a research track that offers a special curriculum for selected students, but Columbia recently moved to a system that encourages all residents to pursue research through a core curriculum and electives. A rich supply of faculty, incentives for mentors, and supportive leadership all have been cited as important ingredients in the success of the above programs. Noted curriculum content includes the usual subjects of biostatistics, research methods, journal clubs, and research management.

Other Aggregate Program Data

Emerging Programs

In an effort to further understand local factors that influence residency-based research training, IOM staff interviewed eight department chairs. These eight chairs were selected because one or more committee members believed their departments were emerging or up-and-coming with regard to interdepartmental research activity. Thus the list of departments selected is representative rather than exhaustive. Furthermore, while these programs appear to be emerging with regard to research activity generally, they have achieved varied success in research training for residents. A list of those interviewed appears in Appendix A.

Unfortunately, these interviews yielded no novel solutions for the research training problem. However, several potential strategies were reinforced by the responses obtained. Specifically, all chairs were asked whether they had any unique strategies for recruiting research-minded residents and faculty. No such strategies were reported. Instead, responses were fairly predictable, with some of the chairs reporting that, while they liked to recruit researchers, research experience was only one of several selection criteria utilized. Several of the chairs noted that research start-up resources were often used as an incentive to attract prospective faculty.

As for research training specifically, all eight department chairs said they had research didactics, six of eight had discretionary funds for research activity, and five said they had a designated faculty member responsible for monitoring research activity within the department (e.g., vice chair for research). Most of the programs had some formal mentoring component, while only four chairs said they had a formal research track, and three said they required residents to take part in research activity.

When asked about obstacles to research training during residency, the majority of chairs stated their belief that limited funding, mentors, and time were key constraints. Nearly all (seven) chairs said that the shortage of child and adolescent psychiatry researchers was especially acute. A majority (six) of the chairs also said that program accreditation requirements limited research training opportunities in residency. However, the perceived magnitude of this limitation was quite variable among the chairs: one felt the requirements enhanced research training, whereas another was vehement that the requirements were inappropriate and excessive. Only one or two chairs believed that any of the following issues were significant barriers to research training in residency: educational debt, competition from Ph.D. investigators, clinical faculty not valuing research, attitude of training director, or lack of interest among residents. Appendix C and Table 4-2 provide some additional detail on the eight emerging programs whose chairs were interviewed, along with other programs reviewed by the committee.

Child Psychiatry Programs

Finally, to understand residency-based research training issues in child and adolescent psychiatry, the committee contacted Robert Hendren, D.O., president of the Society of Professors of Child and Adolescent Psychiatry (SPCAP). SPCAP is a professional society composed of directors of child and adolescent psychiatry programs, many of whom have research experience. Dr. Hendren solicited responses via e-mail from the SPCAP membership to the following questions: (1) Does your institution offer a credible research training course? (2) What would it cost to have a trainee spend 4 hours per week engaged in research training during the 2-year residency program? (3) What would it cost to compensate the "mentor"? and (4) Should research be mandated for trainees? Finally, respondents were asked to state their general opinions about research training and to provide information about where their residents ended up after graduating from the residency program.

Of the 116 child and adolescent training programs represented by SPACP members, Dr. Hendren reported a response rate of 25 percent. Despite that low rate, those who responded appear to represent a reasonable cross section of all programs with regard to size and academic orientation, although other, more obscure response biases remain unknown, making the results potentially idiosyncratic to this subsample. Nevertheless, the results are reported here as at least one window into the structure of child and adolescent psychiatry training.

The responses can be summarized as follows. Nine programs (31 percent) offer courses in research methodology and statistics during residency, although most of those courses are poorly attended. Six additional programs (21 percent) have a more practical course, with either a journal club or some kind of evidence-based teaching. When these courses are associated with food (e.g., if lunch is provided), they are better attended. Regarding the generation of a research product, nine programs (31 percent) require trainees to produce a paper or to present a case at grand rounds. Eight programs (28 percent) were in the process of rethinking their research training didactic at the time of the survey. Respondents have no well-formulated method for evaluating their training program in terms of knowledge gains or research productivity.

Several respondents indicated that there are two main components to the cost of research training: the direct inputs into the training, such as teaching time and equipment/facilities, and the costs associated with losing coverage in the clinics that residents typically staff. Respondents who estimated the costs associated with providing 4 hours per week of research training calculated that doing so would require additional funding of at least $5,000–$10,000 per trainee per year, plus $100 per hour to offset the costs associated with individual mentoring. Divisions with substantial extramural research funding may allow residents to assist with an ongoing study offering direct, but supported, research experience. Even resource-rich divisions, however, may not have the funds to support the ancillary activities (e.g., statistical analysis) required to successfully append a question to an existing research study. Respondents from small programs especially noted the shortage of mentor time as a limiting factor in research training.

Most respondents said that the majority of their trainees did not appear to be interested in research education, basing this conclusion on residents' poor attendance at the research courses offered. Consistent with that evidence, respondents from all levels of programs agreed that research activity in residency should be elective, not mandatory. Furthermore, many respondents suggested that recruiting interested and talented trainees to such research electives was a key challenge that should be addressed with at least two principal strategies. One strategy is to entice junior residents to research training as early as possible in their career, perhaps by formulating an exciting, nationally applicable curriculum in the integrated neural and behavioral sciences. Another strategy is to educate smaller programs about the numerous research training opportunities that exist (e.g., federal and foundation grants, new technology) through seminars, Internet sites, and other outreach methods.

As briefly mentioned in Chapter 3, the principle professional society for child psychiatrists, the American Academy of Child and Adolescent Psychiatry (AACAP) has already made progress in developing model curricula for a "traditional" (i.e., 5-year) residency in adult and child psychiatry and for a 6-year program aimed at "the development of outstanding candidates who are interested in pursuing a career in academic child and adolescent psychiatry" (AACAP, 2003b:2). Both curricula offer a weekly 1.5-hour research seminar beginning in PGY2, research electives of 2 months' duration in PGY3, and research activity beginning in PGY4. For the traditional track, 1 day is set aside for research in PGY4 and 3 days in PGY5. In the 6-year track, 80 percent of time in

PGY5 and PGY6 is dedicated to "mentored research." The program is being developed in collaboration with a number of stakeholders in psychiatry (including the Psychiatry RRC), and it will soon be implemented at Yale University (personal communication, J. Leckman, Yale University, April 4, 2003). Finally, the AACAP curricula are intended to serve as models for programs nationally. Barriers to broad implementation of such curricula include resident stipends beyond PGY4 (see the earlier discussion of GME funding) and the local availability of research mentors and other patient-oriented research resources.

Program Success in Training Researchers

The committee had neither the resources nor the mandate to gather or generate outcome data on a large sample of residency training programs; however, several programs voluntarily provided some limited data indicating the numbers of researchers that have emerged from their training programs. The data are of limited utility because they were not collected in a systematic fashion. Specifically, they do not represent a random sample of programs, and the resulting success rates are not necessarily comparable across programs. Additionally, it should be noted that most programs do not aim to train psychiatrist-researchers, but instead focus on clinical training, so it is unreasonable to expect that a sizable proportion of their trainees will end up on research career paths. Nevertheless, these data are presented in Table 4-2 to offer a summary view of research training rates across *core* residency programs (i.e., not a specialized research track).

Despite the imprecision of the data collected, the numbers in Table 4-2 demonstrate that most residency programs yield career researchers well under 10 percent of the time. The difficulty encountered in obtaining these data—many programs provide only estimates—underscores the fact that residency-based research training is not typically monitored. As expected, the proportion of residents who end up in research careers is well below the proportion of research fellows who do so (see the above descriptions of the Columbia University, WPIC, and University of Michigan programs), again indicating the relevance of postresidency training for psychiatrists truly interested in research.

TABLE 4-2 Research Training Outcome Data from Several Residency Programs in Psychiatry

Psychiatric Residency Program (adult and child together unless noted)	Percentage of Residents Moving into Research[a]	Time Period
Brown University	5.0	1997–2002
Columbia University (adult)	30.0	1985–1999
Duke University (child)	7.5	1992–2002
Emory University	10.0	1997–2002
Indiana University	36.0	1997–2002
Johns Hopkins University (child)	36.0	1997–2002
Medical College of Ohio (child)	0.0	1977–2002
North Dakota University (adult)	0.0	1980–2002
State University of New York–University of Buffalo (child)	0.0	1999–2002
University of Arkansas	12.5	1997–2002
University of Connecticut	10.0	1996–2002
University of Michigan (adult)	19.0	1982–2002
University of Minnesota	10.0	1997–2002
University of Nebraska	2.0	1997–2002
University of Texas at Southwestern	5.0	1997–2002
Neuropsychiatric Institute, University of California, Los Angeles (child)	13.0	1997–2002
Virginia Commonwealth University	5.0	1997–2002
Washington University (adult)	14.0	1998–2002
Washington University (child)	23.0	1992–2002
Western Psychiatric Institute and Clinic	21.0	1996–2001

NOTE: [a]A rough index of the proportion of residents in a given program who move on to research careers. In some cases, this may mean they have been in research careers for several years; in others, it may mean they have recently transitioned to a fellowship or junior research position. *Because these values were not obtained systematically, they are intended only as approximations, not as values for comparison across programs.*

SOURCE: Data were derived from various sources, including correspondence with training directors, website and literature reviews, and eight focused interviews with department chairs. Appendix C offers additional details regarding the programs listed.

A crude comparison of the responses in this table with other research involvement rates among psychiatrists confirm the accuracy of the numbers represented. For example, metafile data from the American Medical Association (AMA) indicate that 2 percent of all practicing psychiatrists in the United States consider research their dominant professional activity (Pasko and Seidman, 2002). Likewise, APA survey data reviewed by economist Douglas Schwalm (2002a; see Chapter 5) indicate that just under 20 percent of psychiatrists engage in any (i.e., greater than 1 percent effort) research activity. Accordingly, meaningful levels of research activity by U.S. psychiatrists likely fall somewhere between 2 and 20 percent, suggesting that the numbers in Table 4-2, which average out to 13 percent, are reasonable, but likely include those who dedicate well under 50 percent of their professional effort to the research endeavor. The data in Table 4-2 may further be used to support the hypothesis that the majority of new researchers in psychiatry are trained at a small number of programs as only 5 of the 20 programs represented claimed that 20 percent or more of their residents moved into research careers.

CONCLUSIONS AND RECOMMENDATIONS

This chapter has described institutional, departmental, and curricular factors that influence research training in residency. Funding, mentoring, and resident scheduling issues appear to be the chief constraints on research training in residency. Funding for residency training is heavily influenced by Medicare GME policies, and that funding stream is under increasing negative pressure. Research is not generally considered part of core residency training. As a result, funding for research activity needs to be justified independently and obtained either from extramural grants or from discretionary internal funds (e.g., endowments, profits from practice plans). Leaders of medical institutions have control over how Medicare and other funds are distributed. They additionally set expectations regarding trainee and faculty activities through organizational systems, such as those that determine promotional policies and general resource allocation. Accordingly, leaders (e.g., department chairs, deans, presidents) play a key role in assigning value to and maintaining the research mission, which includes research didactics and activity within training programs. Therefore, the committee believes the following recommendation is critical to research training in psychiatry:

Recommendation 4.1. The broad psychiatry community should work more aggressively to encourage uni-

versity presidents, deans and hospital chief executive officers to give greater priority to the advancement of mental health through investments in leadership, faculty, and infrastructure for research and research training in psychiatry departments.

Although this recommendation applies equally to most branches of medical research, psychiatric research is arguably of particular importance in this regard. This is the case because current opportunities in brain and behavioral research are so great (see Chapter 1), and because mental illness is the object of considerable stigma that appears to have the dual effects of inhibiting efficient health care delivery (e.g., getting patients to the doctor), and impeding full reimbursement for rendered mental health services. The Surgeon General's Report on Mental Health demonstrates as well as any document the relative importance of mental health; the ways in which the brain and behavioral sciences have advanced in recent years and the relevance of future advances to overall health; and the extent to which deeply engrained stigma works against equitable funding for mental health care—inequities that adversely affect research advances, which are partially subsidized by clinical revenues (DHHS, 1999).

Accordingly, medical administrators should be aggressively encouraged to invest in expanding research training in psychiatry as a first step to at least bring psychiatrists on par with the research efforts of many other medical specialists (e.g., subspecialties of internal medicine, neurology). Department chairs and other leaders can promote psychiatric research by developing and financing a long-term business plan that considers the monetary, marketing, and societal benefits likely to result from mental health research. Institutional executives need to be encouraged to invest in these plans by utilizing reasonable portions of their general funds (e.g., IME, dean's tax, endowments) and by frequently including psychiatric research agendas in fund-raising efforts. At the same time, these leaders (especially those in psychiatry) should educate medical students and residents regarding the extraordinary intellectual ventures that accompany research in psychiatry. To the extent that such education and promotion efforts are already occurring, it is the committee's sense that they need to be expanded if any real gains are to be made in the number of psychiatry trainees tracking to research careers.

One of the most intensive forms of leadership is mentoring. Mentoring is probably the ingredient cited most frequently as necessary for effective research training. The shortage of mentors is also a commonly noted barrier to effective research training. Accordingly, the committee believes that financial incentives may be important to encourage more senior researchers, particularly at small institutions, to enter the mentoring pool. Accordingly, the committee makes the following recommendation:

> **Recommendation 4.2. Academic institutions and their psychiatry residency training programs should reward the involvement of patient-oriented research faculty in the residency training process. The National Institute of Mental Health should take the lead in identifying funding mechanisms to support such incentives.**

This recommendation targets in particular smaller institutions with limited resources to offer a broad range of research experiences to and mentors for their trainees. Trainees in well-established programs are more likely to "pay for themselves" by extending the productivity of the mentor, and supplements to existing grants can be used to cover some of the costs associated with the trainees' work. At less resource-intensive institutions, however, prospective trainees will likely be less familiar with research methods so that mentoring will require a greater investment of time with a potentially lower return in terms of trainee productivity. In these contexts, the committee encourages mechanisms to finance mentoring, with the provision that grant renewal would depend on the research success of the mentor's past trainees. As an alternative to on-site mentoring, a remote system of mentoring might be devised to give both faculty and trainees the opportunity to be matched with individuals having similar interests outside of their institution. Furthermore, such a network might be sustained by offering senior mentors consulting fees or other remunerative support (e.g., travel, equipment) for their expertise and time.

In addition to issues related to institutional leadership and mentoring, this chapter has reviewed clinical research training programs generally and several psychiatry residency programs with regard to research training. The programs reviewed are highly variable. For example, nonpsychiatry training includes clinical research programs that range from 1-year certificates to multiyear programs culminating with a Ph.D. Although this range appears to be geared in part to the broad range of applicants, an AAMC task force concluded that program variability reflects imprecision regarding the formal constitution of clinical research training. Research training in psychiatric residency is also variable. Nevertheless, common best practices are apparent from reviewing existing programs and published descriptions. Most programs offer research training in the latter years of residency, and even the most research-intensive institutions route their research-oriented graduates toward additional training, usually in the form of a fellowship. Hands-on activity in residency is encouraged when resources and mentoring are available. Key course subject matter includes epidemiology, grant and manuscript writing, design of clinical trials, and research ethics.

Unfortunately, little has been done to integrate research training into all or even most of the residency years. Additionally, existing curricula are not typically validated by careful long-term follow-up studies to determine whether trainees actually were encouraged to move into patient-oriented research careers, or toward more evidence-based practice methods. Therefore, the committee makes the following recommendation:

> **Recommendation 4.3. The National Institute of Mental Health, foundations, and other funding agencies should provide resources to support efforts to create competency-based curricula for research literacy and more comprehensive research training in psychiatry that are applicable across the spectrum of adult (general) and child and adolescent residency training programs. Supported curriculum development efforts should include plans for educating faculty to deliver each new curriculum, as well as plans for evaluating each curriculum's success in training individuals to competency and in recruiting and training successful researchers.**

On the federal level, the K30 mechanism is an obvious means of supporting some curriculum development, although it does not have provisions for stipend support and is rarely utilized by medical residents. The AACAP research pathways are, to the committee's knowledge, among the best models generated to date for creating and evaluating an exportable model for training psychiatrist-researchers, in this case targeting those in child and adolescent psychiatry. Such efforts should be extended to various other settings, including resource-poor departments and those that emphasize a given subspecialty of psychiatric practice (e.g., psychotherapy, addiction, pain management). These curricula should be aimed at sparking residents' interest in a lifelong career in patient-oriented research without interfering with core clinical training. The principal aim of this recommendation, however, is to ensure that all residents are adequately introduced to the concepts of research and that research training is not merely an afterthought to residency education. Thus the recommendation is focused on ensuring a foundation in the residency curriculum for patient-oriented research efforts. Even residents who intend to become clinicians should be introduced to the concepts and findings of patient-oriented research as a necessary complement to their clinical training. Curricula should be developed using established educational principles; it is especially important to include evaluation phases to verify the utility of the curricula in the training of patient-oriented psychiatrist-researchers and evidence-based practitioners (Sheets and Anderson, 1991). Novel ways to integrate research training into the residency experience for future clinicians and the next generation of independent investigators should also be considered. For example, Duke University is currently experimenting with a program that introduces research activity in PGY1 rather than waiting until later in the residency (list serve communication,[29] G. Thrall, Duke University, January 12, 2003).

With regard to curriculum development, the committee believes that, since psychiatric training programs vary considerably in terms of size and local expertise, they should be viewed along a hierarchical research training continuum that ranges from those providing only research literacy to those training large numbers of patient-oriented psychiatrist-researchers. The committee proposes such a continuum in Table 4-3 (see page 131). An important feature of this continuum is the detail it provides about program components (e.g., longitudinal participation in research) and the corresponding department infrastructure (e.g., mentors and existing grants) necessary to achieve various levels of research training.

The schema represented in Table 4-3 shows how individual programs can consider their current infrastructure and build on their clinical and research strengths to enhance research training. For example, the presence of a large substance abuse clinic could be used as the foundation for a grant application to establish a research or research training effort in substance abuse, thereby advancing the program along the research training continuum. The continuum additionally is intended as a tool that can be used to implement the following recommendation:

> **Recommendation 4.4. The National Institute of Mental Health should support those departments that are poised to improve their residency-based research training to achieve measurable increases in patient-oriented research careers among their trainees. Support for such programs should include funds to:**

---

[29] The list serve is maintained by the AADPRT.

- Hire faculty and staff dedicated to research and research training efforts.
- Acquire equipment and enhance facilities for research training.
- Initiate pilot and/or short-term research activities for residents.
- Educate adult and child and adolescent residency training directors and other faculty in how to promote and guide research career planning.

This recommendation aims to encourage NIMH to enhance the resources and environment of programs that can realistically advance their training efforts to the next level on the research continuum set forth in Table 4-3. A request for applications would best call for proposals from across the continuum, with the aim of funding a few programs at each of the three delineated levels (i.e., purely clinical, moderate research training, superior research training). Review committees for such grants would be instructed to rank applications on the basis of each program's ability to demonstrate a plan for moving to and sustaining a higher lever of research training. At the bottom end of the continuum, programs would be expected to instill research literacy in their residents. Programs would also be expected to encourage their residents to transfer to other institutions (after 3-years of training) and aim for research fellowships to optimize their research training; for weaker programs, some altruism would be required if they did not have the local infrastructure to support a promising trainee.

Regarding the details of this recommendation, the first three bullets listed are linked quite directly to developing a research infrastructure. NIH or other agency grants—similar to the General Clinical Research Center or Biomedical Research Infrastructure Network grants—might be useful to this end. The expired Research Infrastructure Support Program (RISP), which still exists to help minority-based programs develop a foundation (see Chapter 5), is clearly a direct model for what is implied by this recommendation. The RISP was "...designed to enable institutions with relatively small but viable research programs...to develop into significantly stronger...research settings" (NIMH, 1994:2). That mechanism included possible support for: salaries, research training for junior investigators, and research instruments/equipment. One current RISP program announcement calls for applications for the funding of mental health services research at primarily clinical facilities. An important component of that announcement is that small programs are encouraged

Table 4-3 Continuum of Residency-Based Research Training

Level[a]	Program Components	Required Department Infrastructure	Notes
Solid research "track" (center of excellence[b])	• 3 years core and 3 years research training • Strong connectivity between residency and post-residency research training • Residents aim for career (K) and a research (R) grant submission and a career in research • All components listed below	• Strong research culture/leadership • Expertise in several disciplines • Administrative support • Dedicated research resources • Research committee • Liaison with relevant facilities • Research training grants • Multiple major grants • Rich supply of mentors	• For research-oriented M.D.'s and M.D./Ph.D.'s • Program should be principal source of career patient-oriented researchers
Provision of research experience	• Coursework emphasizing methods and statistics • Longitudinal participation in a research project • Scholarly product • All components listed below	• Research culture • Research residency training director • Research funds • At least three major grants (e.g., R01's) • Available mentors	• Those interested in research careers should be encouraged to transfer to a "center of excellence" after 3 years of core training
Training of research-literate residents	• Coursework • Seminars • Grand rounds • Research rounds • Journal club • Visiting lectureships • Informatics[c]	• Minimal research • Few mentors	• Psychiatry Residency Review Committee should mandate this for all programs • Foundation for evidence-based practice • Graduates should be able to assimilate scientific literature into clinical practice • Those interested in research careers should be encouraged to transfer to a more research-intensive program after 3 years of core training

← Continuum

[a] Most research-intensive program is listed at the top.
[b] Some information from David Kupfer interview in Meyer and McLaughlin, 1998.
[c] Knowledge about how to obtain, electronically archive, and efficiently review, the latest in data germane to mental health research and practice.

to develop direct collaborations with research-intensive institutions (NIMH, 2000c). This and other similar programs should be developed to improve research education at psychiatry training facilities.

With regard to bullet number 3 under recommendation 4.4, pilot or short-term funding could be utilized opportunistically by departments to facilitate the inclusion of more residents in research training. This is the case because residency is typically a career phase that permits limited and transient opportunities for the pursuit of nonclinical interests. A modest, but available pool of pilot funding might be used to support one or more training slots or other research-related resources to accommodate qualified and motivated residents.

The final item listed under recommendation 4.4 addresses the need to provide training directors and faculty with adequate instruction in guiding and nurturing potential researchers. Models at NIMH already exist in the form of seminars for K awardees (Tuma et al., 1987). Similar "retreats" for residency training directors and/or vice chairs of research could facilitate the flow of information on research training grants and other relevant matters to those most responsible for training residents. This recommendation also encourages the expansion and utilization of other means of information dissemination. These mechanisms include web-based resources, such as the NIH K Kiosk, which allows one to search and review various mentored career awards (NIH, 2003e). They further include on-line tutorials, such as one that currently exists on protecting the rights of research subjects (NIH, 2003f).

5

Personal Factors

The last two chapters focused on external factors that impact on a resident's decision to pursue research training. This chapter turns to more intrinsic or personal factors that influence such career choices. It briefly reviews innate characteristics that correlate with the decision to pursue a research career, and then personal financial issues that impact on research career initiation and development. Finally, it addresses gender, racial, and ethnic issues as factors relevant to training major subsets of psychiatric trainees. Included is a discussion of issues faced by foreign medical graduates who matriculate into psychiatric residency programs in the United States. The chapter ends with conclusions and recommendations.

INNATE CHARACTERISTICS

Several key personal characteristics correlate with the decision to pursue a research career. They include motivation and drive, and intellectual capacity and scientific orientation.

Motivation and Drive

Some of the personal factors that move one to pursue a research career transcend or precede formal medical educational experiences. Motivation and drive, or rationale and persistence, are certainly relevant in the pursuit of any complex goal. Formal education and mentoring may have some impact on these characteristics, but other, less tangible and less malleable factors are likely to be relevant, if not dominant.

Personal experiences that motivate one toward a research career include direct or familial experience with mental illness. Such is the case for genetics researcher Edwin Cook who said, "I do [autism research] because…I always wanted to know what was wrong with my brother and to help him…." (National Public Radio, 2002). Alternatively, one may have extraordinary curiosity and skill that lead to a productive research career despite the absence of direct support and encouragement in the context of formal medical training. This was the case with Eric Kandel (1998), a psychiatrist and Nobel Prize winner for his neuroscience work, who recently wrote that his psychiatric residency involved very little scholarly activity and virtually no research training. Despite these omissions from his training, he and many of his peers went on to become successful basic and patient-oriented researchers, evidence that skilled researchers can emerge from residency programs with little or no research training.

These examples are presented as a reminder of two principles. First, certain characteristics that correlate with research productivity are difficult if not impossible to shape in the context of formal medical training. Second, it is wise for any field to identify, support, and attempt to attract the brightest and most driven candidates, and to encourage them to pursue a career aimed at critiquing and expanding that discipline's knowledge base.

Intellectual Capacity and Scientific Orientation

In addition to motivation and drive, intellectual capacity and scientific orientation are logically correlated with research productivity. Research requires the ability to master an existing and constantly expanding knowledge base, and to formulate and test new ideas in an effort to clarify, broaden, or even revise what is known about the subject under study. Additionally, research productivity is dependent upon regular and detailed oral and written communications with peers as a key means of validating the accuracy and relevance of an experiment or theory. In psychiatric research, it is reasonable to assume that such skills correlate, at least partially, with scores on standardized tests used to evaluate applicants to medical school (Medical College Admission Test [MCAT]) or to verify that medical students and graduates are prepared for independent practice (U.S. Medical Licensing Examination [USMLE]). To the extent that these proxies for research aptitude are valid, there is some indication that the discipline of psychiatry may not be attracting the brightest students, and from this one can infer that inadequate recruitment of the brightest students may negatively impact on psychiatry's ability to expand its ranks of patient-oriented researchers.

Sierles and Taylor (1995) reviewed literature on medical students' interest in psychiatry and found that, as of the late 1980s, those favoring psychiatry tended to have relatively low science scores compared with their peers who were interested in other medical specialties. A more recent review of MCAT and USMLE scores by economist Sean Nicholson of the Wharton Business School further supports that conclusion (Arcidiacono and Nicholson, Unpublished; Nicholson, 2002). Nicholson's findings are based on 1996–1998 survey and exam score data from the National Board of Medical Examiners for approximately 33,000 medical school students. Nicholson found that fourth-year medical students who chose psychiatry as their specialty had the lowest average scores on their preclinical USMLE (Step 1, a measure of basic medical science knowledge) compared with those selecting 15 other specialties (see Table 5-1). He also found that those aiming to pursue a career in psychiatry upon entering medical school ranked ninth on the MCAT. The higher ranking of these students on the MCAT may be related to the fact that this test includes more verbal/social science content than the USMLE, or that some of the more successful test takers favoring psychiatry in the first year of medical school changed their specialty selection 3 years later at the time of the USMLE (see Table 5-1). What is not clear from Nicholson's analysis is whether the apparent differences in exam scores represent normally distributed samples of training physicians or the distributions are multimodal (e.g., those choosing psychiatry may be composed of one group with relatively high scores and another group with relatively low scores). Additionally, Nicholson's analysis is limited because 30 percent of the universe of more than 47,000 medical graduates from 1996–1998 did not complete one of the surveys or otherwise had incomplete data records (Arcidiacono and Nicholson, Unpublished). Accordingly, the analysis is incomplete; nonetheless it represents the best comparison of early and later training examination scores that the committee was able to identify for this report.

TABLE 5-1 Examination Scores by Specialty Choice upon Entry to Medical School (MCAT) and upon Entry to Residency (USMLE)

Specialty Choice[a]	Mean MCAT Score (rank)	Mean USMLE (Step 1) Score (rank)
Ear, Nose, and Throat (ENT)	28.4 (5)	224.4 (1)
Dermatology	26.6 (17)	219.2 (2)
Surgical Subspecialty	28.6 (3)	218.4 (3)
Orthopedic Surgery	28.4 (5)	218.1 (4)
Urology	27.5 (14)	215.7 (5)
Radiology	28.7 (2)	213.8 (6)
General Surgery	28.3 (7)	213.4 (7)
Ophthalmology	28.0 (9)	213.4 (7)
Pathology	27.6 (12)	213.3 (9)
Internal Medicine	28.5 (4)	212.3 (10)
Emergency Medicine	28.1 (8)	211.4 (11)
Obstetrics-Gynecology (OB-GYN)	27.1 (15)	208.1 (12)
Pediatrics	27.6 (12)	207.4 (13)
Anesthesiology	27.1 (15)	206.8 (14)
Family Practice	27.8 (11)	204.8 (15)
Psychiatry	28.0 (9)	204.2 (16)
Undecided	28.8 (1)	N/A
Total	28.2	210.5

NOTES: Data are from 33,110 medical students who graduated from medical school from 1996 to 1998. The sample represents a subset of more than 47,000 graduates during that time period. Individuals were excluded because of missing data or because they refused to consent to having their information used for research purposes. MCAT = Medical College Admission Test; USMLE = U.S. Medical Licensing Examination; N/A = not available.
[a]Choice when polled at 1st year of medical school with respect to MCAT scores, and at 4th year of medical school with respect to USMLE scores.
SOURCE: Arcidiacono and Nicholson (Unpublished), Nicholson (2002).

Using 1992 Association of American Medical Colleges (AAMC) survey data, Nicholson also found that medical students who considered research an important factor in determining their choice of medical specialty had higher MCAT scores than those who did not consider research an important factor. In further support of the link between MCAT scores and research aspirations, albeit without any statistical validation, data from a 1994 questionnaire on over 10,000 medical school graduates showed that the more than 1,000 individuals with research interests had higher science scores (mean = 10.32) on their MCAT than their colleagues who were uninterested in research (mean = 9.22) (Kassebaum et al., 1995). These data fall well short of full confirmation that high standardized test scores on either the MCAT or USMLE correlate with successful patient-oriented research careers, but they do support the concern expressed by some in psychiatry that the discipline is currently not attracting the brightest medical students (Hyman, 2002b; Meyer, 2002).

In addition to attracting applicants with somewhat lower scientific aptitudes than other branches of medicine, psychiatry has historically attracted those with a predisposition for the social sciences and humanities (Fishman and Zimet, 1972; Lee et al., 1995; Nemetz and Weiner, 1965; Paiva and Haley, 1971). This view was reinforced by John March, Director of Programs in Child and Adolescent Anxiety Disorders and Developmental Psychopharmacology, Duke University, who said in his presentation at the committee's workshop:

> Psychiatry has a very strong humanistic culture...unlike the rest of medicine, which has gotten very technological....So you find folks that are drawn to psychiatry who don't have the kind of minds that tend to like scientific reductionistic reasoning (March, 2002).

This apparent recruitment bias is, in certain ways, good for patient-oriented research as it likely enhances the doctor–patient relationship. However, there is also evidence that some medical students avoid psychiatry because they believe it is a discipline with a limited scientific basis (Feifel et al., 1999). This latter issue may be linked to psychiatry's difficulty in attracting medical students with the scientific orientation necessary to function as successful biomedical researchers. Difficulties in recruiting and retaining individuals in the field may also be the result of the stigma society attaches to mental illness and persons with mental illness. It is reasonable to assume that medical students may harbor some of these same negative perceptions about people with mental illness and about the medical professionals who treat them. For example, a 2001 survey of second-year medical students at the University of Arkansas found that more than 30 percent believed electroconvulsive therapy (ECT) was used as a form of punishment, and 40 percent believed psychiatrists did not use ECT appropriately (Clothier et al., 2001). This rather dramatic misperception is in stark contrast to the realities of ECT (U. S. Department of Health and Human Services [DHHS], 1999).

Furthermore, psychiatry has long been a profession for which cultural stereotypes abound, and most of those stereotypes are not altogether positive. As discussed in Chapter 4, psychiatrists engaged in patient-oriented research are underinvolved in medical student and resident education. Therefore, medical students' exposure to psychiatrists frequently does not include exposure to psychiatrists doing exciting research that addresses intellectually challenging, interesting, and clinically relevant issues. The media frequently depict mental health professionals in general and psychiatrists in particular as inept or eccentric, rather than bright, well-trained medical professionals who are addressing extremely important health care issues (British Broadcasting Company, 2002). Clearly, one way to redress this negative stereotyping is to ensure that medical students are exposed to the best and brightest psychiatry has to offer, including successful patient-oriented researchers.

PERSONAL FINANCIAL CONCERNS

Quite apart from the innate characteristics discussed above, medical students and psychiatric residents have financial concerns that intensify as they progress through their training. This section describes those concerns as they pertain to entry into residency and possible pursuit of a research career.

Student Debt

Trainees incur substantial educational debt while in medical school. In 2002, the cost of attending a public medical school averaged nearly $28,000 per year, while that of attending a private medical school averaged $44,000 (AAMC, 2002c). Data from 2000 to 2002 indicate that over 80 percent of medical students take out loans to finance their medical education (AAMC, 2002c). In 2002, average debt among medical school graduates stood at $104,000 (AAMC, 2002b; 2002c; Sung et al., 2003). After adjusting for inflation, the median level of debt for medical school graduates doubled between 1985 and 1998 (Proctor, 2000; Zemlo et al., 2000).

Further investigation supports the hypothesis that debt load has an impact on career decisions. Data from the early 1990s, for example, demonstrate that medical students with high debt favored high-paying specialties over primary care disciplines (e.g., pediatrics and family medicine) (Berg et al., 1993; Colquitt et al., 1996). Given that mean salaries for psychiatrists fall in a range comparable to that for the primary care specialties (AAMC, 2002b; Bureau of Labor Statistics, 2002; Nicholson, 2002), it is plausible that students with high debt will avoid psychiatry in favor of a more lucrative specialty so they can repay their educational debt more easily (see the discussion below).

Residency and Fellowship Stipends

Compensation for residents and fellows is low in comparison with entry-level salaries. Data for 2002 from New York State place entry-level salaries for new graduates of psychiatric residencies at $124,000 and $144,000 for adult and for child and adolescent psychiatrists, respectively (Nolan et al., 2003). In comparison, first-year postgraduate (PGY1) residents at Columbia University earn $43,000, and research fellows (PGY5 to PGY8) receive stipends of approximately $75,000 (personal communication, R. Rieder, Columbia University, March 31, 2003). Since New York State supplements Medicare graduate medical education funds with state funds, other regions where state support is not available will likely compensate residents at even lower levels. The shortest core residency training period accredited by the Accreditation Council for Graduate Medical Education (ACGME) is 3 years (e.g., general internal medicine, pediatrics). Additional residency or research fellowship training beyond that point is not necessary for core certification (e.g., to take the psychiatry boards), but rather requires extended training and only sometimes yields additional certification. Thus, a recent medical school graduate may weigh the value of additional training against the short-term loss in income that is represented by differences between training stipends and entry-level salaries, differences that can dissuade a new physician from pursuing psychiatry or research training.

Salaries of Psychiatrists Compared with Other Specialties

Psychiatrists, especially child and adolescent psychiatrists, earn less than many other medical specialists with similar post–medical school training periods (see Table 5-2), although it is notable that among 4-year residencies, pathologists start at lower salaries than those of adult psychiatrists. Among 5-year residencies, child and adolescent psychiatrists have lower starting salaries than urologists, general surgeons, radiologists, and orthopedic surgeons. Overall salary structure does not favor psychiatry ov-

TABLE 5-2 Median Expected Starting Income for Graduates of New York State and California Residency Training Programs, 2002

Specialty	Minimum Number of Years of Postgraduate Medical Education	Median Expected Salary (2002) (thousands of dollars)	
		New York	California
Anesthesiology	4	194	206
Dermatology	4	155	148
Ophthalmology	4	133	137
Neurology	4	126	138
Adult Psychiatry	4	**124**	**120**
Pathology	4	118	112
Orthopedics	5	225	208
Radiology	5	218	198
General Surgery	5	157	164
Urology	5	155	206
Child Psychiatry	5	**144**	**140**

SOURCE: ACGME (2002a), Nolan et al. (2003).

er many other medical disciplines, a reality that appears to influence career decisions.

To further understand the impact of income expectations and salary on an individual's choice of specialty, the committee again turned to the work of Sean Nicholson at the Wharton School of Business. Using 1992 data from the National Residency Matching Program (NRMP) and the AAMC, Nicholson (2002b) considered how specialty selection is influenced by specialty income. He found a direct and significant correlation between specialty income and relative demand for a given specialty among medical students.[30] Figure 5-1 summarizes this finding graphically. What is apparent from this graph and from the evidence presented

---

[30]Relative demand for a given specialty is defined as the ratio of the number of graduating medical students selecting a specialty as their first choice, divided by the total number of national slots available in that specialty.

above is that psychiatry is one of the lowest-paying specialties in medicine, and that this relatively low compensation may impact negatively on recruitment to the discipline's residency. At the same time, income correlations alone likely oversimplify the importance of economics to medical students selecting a specialty. A 2003 study found that medical students were apt to consider specialties based on, from most to least important, expected annual work hours, length of residency training, weekly hours worked, and earnings (Thornton and Esposto, 2003). Thus it appears that medical students value time as well as money.

Salary Differences Between Clinicians and Researchers

In addition to high student debt, low stipends during residency and fellowship, and lower salaries in comparison with those of other medical specialties, psychiatry trainees interested in research may face the possi-

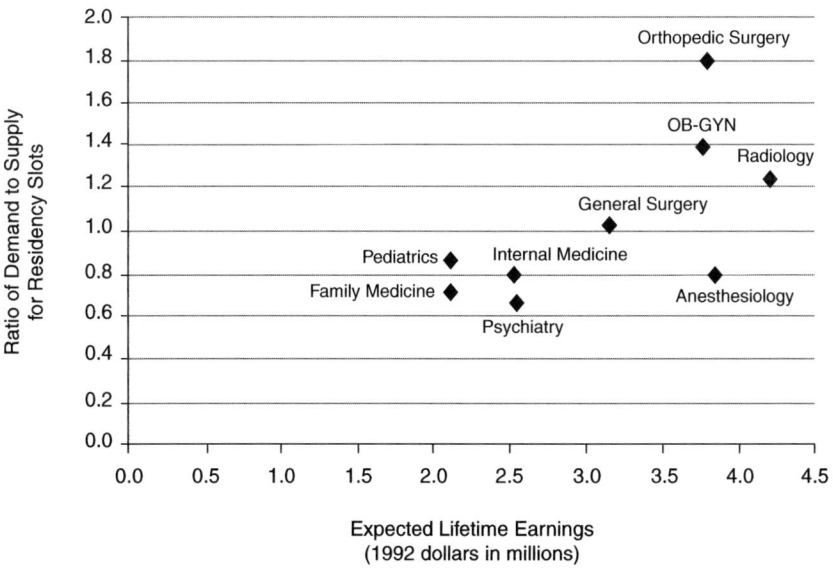

FIGURE 5-1 Ratio of demand to supply of medical students who designate a given residency as their first career choice, versus the expected lifetime income of that residency. Based on 1992 National Residency Matching data for 14,030 U.S. medical graduates. Supply is the total number of national slots available in that specialty.
SOURCE: Data from Nicholson (2002).

bility that they will not receive the same compensation as their clinician counterparts. There appears to be no published literature on the salary differences between psychiatrists who are researchers and those who are clinicians. However, the committee was able to find published data comparing the salaries of researchers and clinicians in psychology. In a 2001 survey of members of the American Psychological Association, the mean salary for new[31] doctoral-level psychologists who rated themselves as full-time researchers (both basic and clinical) and who were not faculty at academic institutions was $58,000 (n = 126).[32] For new[31] clinically-licensed psychologists who claimed direct mental health care as their primary activity and who also were not based at an academic institution (n = 175), the mean salary was $63,500.[32] For faculty at academic institutions, both researchers and non-researchers, with the rank of lecturer, instructor, and assistant professor (n=599), the mean salary was $61,000 (Singleton et al., 2003).[32] Although this survey did not isolate clinical or other psychologists engaged in part-time research, nor does it permit full adjustments for years of professional experience, the data support the hypothesis that psychologists engaged predominantly in research, at least in their early professional years, earn lower base salaries than their clinician counterparts. It is plausible that this salary differential extends to other clinical behavioral disciplines, such as psychiatry.

To consider psychiatrists directly, the committee commissioned the work of economist Douglas Schwalm of Louisiana State University, as his dissertation (2002b) focused on the impact of managed care and research activity on psychiatrists' incomes. At the request of the committee, Schwalm (2002a) adjusted his analysis to consider specifically the impact of research involvement on those incomes. He examined data from the 1998 National Survey of Psychiatric Practice, conducted by the American Psychiatric Association (APA). Of the 1,500 APA member psychiatrists surveyed in that year, 1,076 responded, and 628 provided annual income information. Of the subsample providing annual income data, 112 (18 percent) reported some involvement in research activities; these included 26 female respondents.[33] The basic statistical model regressed the log-income to a quadratic of years of experience, gender, research, and work setting.[34] After removing the effect of work setting,

---

[31] "New" is defined as having 0 to 9 years experience

[32] Salary extrapolated to 12-month equivalent.

[33] Psychiatrists were considered researchers if they self-reported themselves as such and if they spent any time in research (i.e., no minimal cut-off was used to define a researcher).

[34] Such log-income regression models are based on the human capital model devised by Gary Becker, which has been used extensively to estimate the effects of several factors, including income, on career choice (Becker, 1993; Mincer, 1974).

which is nonsignificant, and adjusting for the significant effects of years of experience and gender, Schwalm found that on average, psychiatrist-researchers earn approximately 20 percent less than their nonresearcher counterparts. Assuming a retirement age of 70, this loss of income translates to a reduction in lifetime earnings of $600,000 to $1 million (1998 dollars). For women, the annual salary difference between researchers and nonresearchers is negligible; however, the extrapolated hourly wage favors female clinicians over researchers (see Table 5-3). The modeling results further indicate that, while psychiatrists who spend *any* (i.e., greater than 1 percent) of their time engaged in research activities earn less than their full-time clinician counterparts, psychiatrists who devote more than 20 percent of their time to research earn more than those who spend a smaller proportion of their time engaged in research activities, although their salary never recovers to the level of full-time clinicians.

There are two key limitations to the above analysis. First, researchers in this dataset are disproportionately at academic institutions (e.g., medical schools), and thus their salaries are likely lower in part because of

TABLE 5-3 Selected Data from the American Psychiatric Association's 1998 National Survey of Psychiatric Practice

Full-Time Employed Psychiatrists (n = 628[a])	Males	Females
Nonresearcher Annual Salary	$143,000[c]	$111,000
Researcher Annual Salary	$121,000	$114,000
Nonresearcher Hours Worked[b]	52	44
Researcher Hours Worked[b]	56	51
Nonresearcher-Implicit Wage[d]	$55/hour	$50/hour
Researcher-Implicit Wage[d]	$43/hour	$45/hour

[a]Of these respondents, 112 had spent some time as researchers, including 26 females and 31 non-Caucasians.
[b]Respondents gave the number of hours they worked in the week prior to the time at which they completed the survey.
[c]Significantly different from male researchers (p $\leq$ 0.01).
[d]Implicit wage = annual salary/(hours of work × 50).
SOURCE: Data adapted from Schwalm (2002a).

their practice location.[35] Second, the dataset includes very few respondents who considered research their primary activity or who spent at least 40 percent of their time engaged in research. Thus it is not known whether those who spend more than 40 percent of their time in research earn lower salaries than those of their clinician colleagues. Nevertheless, the data suggest that psychiatrist-researchers earn less and work longer hours than psychiatrist-clinicians (see Table 5-3).

Nonsalary Benefits of a Research Career

Given the combination of high educational debt, low training stipends, and relatively low salaries for psychiatrists and psychiatrist-researchers, it is no surprise that financial issues may well dissuade some from the latter career. Nevertheless, there are many nonfinancial reasons to choose a career in biomedical and psychiatric research. Therefore, in addition to educating prospective researchers about the challenges they may face, the committee believes it equally important to educate psychiatrist trainees about the potential nonsalary benefits of a career in mental health research. Those nonsalary benefits are enumerated in Box 5-1 and briefly described in the following text.

BOX 5-1

Nonsalary Benefits of a Research Career

- Excitement of discovery
- Variety of activities and flexible schedule
- Broad network of colleagues and international travel
- Consulting to industry/government/foundations
- Innovative and leading-edge techniques
- Competitiveness of psychiatrists applying for grant funding

---

[35]Schwalm reviewed American Medical Association data from 1997 and found that individuals in academic settings (researchers and others) typically earn 11 to 17 percent less than those working in other settings (e.g., private offices).

Excitement of Discovery

The experience of discovery, of being the first to understand or validate a small piece of the universe, can be quite extraordinary. In the words of chemist and Nobel laureate Max Perutz, "Making a discovery is such a wonderful thing. It's like falling in love and getting to the top of a mountain all in one" (Rosenberg, 2002:368). Given the brain's importance in governing human physiology and thought, it is not an overstatement to say that research in the treatment and prevention of mental illness addresses some of the most complex and intriguing topics faced by contemporary patient-oriented researchers. A demonstration of the complexity of this research and its central importance to medical science comes from leaders in the field of genetics. James Watson, co-discoverer of the double helix structure of DNA and one of the initiators of the Human Genome Project in 1986, recently said:

> Driving me in 1986 was the slow and painful realization that we had a son with a very disturbed and non-functional mind. And I thought we probably never will understand why Rufus is sick until we get the genetic causation of mental disease. So I wanted to [initiate the Human Genome Project as soon as possible]. (National Public Radio, 2003)

Commenting on the complexity of the underpinnings of mental disorders, Aravinda Chakravarti, Director of The Johns Hopkins University's Institute of Genetic Medicine, said:

> Environmental influences and other aspects of our diet and lifestyle clearly also impact on the functioning of these genes, and exactly how that affects the functioning of this very complex organism [sic] called the brain is clearly one of the great mysteries. (National Public Radio, 2003)

Variety of Activities and Flexible Work Schedule

Research often permits one to engage in a variety of activities that provide substantial and beneficial respite from the potential tedium and stress of day-to-day patient care responsibilities. Patient-oriented research offers the opportunity to grapple inventively with otherwise intractable problems that can induce professional frustration and burnout, such as treatment-resistant disorders. Additionally, although research activities are intense, they can be less time-critical than acute patient care, thereby yielding a more flexible work schedule than is possible with a full-time clinical load. Research work that requires considerable reading and writing can furthermore be carried out at home or on travel as it is not necessarily tied to a clinical or inpatient unit. Although the committee was unable to find time-use studies confirming whether researchers work more hours than their clinical colleagues, data from the National Survey of Psychiatric Practice analyzed by Schwalm (see Table 5-3 above) indicate that researchers in psychiatry work more hours than their clinician counterparts. Future studies are needed to validate this apparent increased time commitment and to determine whether more time engaged in work corresponds with higher occupational burden or greater job satisfaction.

Broad Network of Colleagues

Research careers foster the development of a broad network of colleagues both within and outside the discipline of psychiatry, many of whom are likely to add new dimensions and perspectives to the work of academic psychiatrists. Multidisciplinary efforts have become essential to scientific programs across the brain and behavioral sciences (IOM, 2000). Networks established with colleagues at one's home university, as well as nationally and internationally, provide potential sources of personal and professional satisfaction. These connections also can result in opportunities to make presentations, serve as a visiting scholar, or take on an advisory role. Because they are constantly working on cutting-edge techniques (see below), successful psychiatrist-researchers often are invited to serve as consultants to government and to drug and biotechnology companies. In this capacity, they can influence the development of new psychiatric treatments that may substantially increase the nation's mental health, and, with due diligence to avoid potential conflicts of interest, can also increase their own personal income through consulting fees.

Innovative and Leading-Edge Techniques

Patient-oriented research allows academic faculty members not only to practice innovatively, but also to generate leading-edge techniques and to influence the direction of the field of behavioral medicine. Psychiatrist-researcher Peter McGuffin, for example, believes his work has been a factor in encouraging mainstream psychiatry to accept the importance of genetic research for understanding the causes of many psychiatric disorders (ISI Thomson, 2001b). Kenneth Davis, also a well-established psychiatrist-researcher, believes some of his efforts have helped shift research in schizophrenia from a focus on hallucinations and delusions to one aimed more broadly at abnormalities in cognition (ISI Thomson, 2001a).

Competitiveness of Psychiatrists Applying for Grant Funding

In addition to financial factors that influence a medical student's decision regarding a career in psychiatric research, the committee believes strongly that potential psychiatrist-researchers are concerned about their prospects for obtaining grant funding throughout their career. The prospect of competing for soft money on a regular basis, in addition to publishing or perishing, is a daunting one and clearly represents a key barrier to many considering a research career. Nevertheless, there is considerable evidence to suggest that when they apply, M.D.'s are as successful as Ph.D.'s at obtaining federal research funds. This point is significant because it is well known that most Ph.D. programs, such as those training clinical psychologists, include far more training in research methodology than do medical school programs (IOM, 1994). Furthermore, a high proportion of Ph.D. students aim toward academic careers, whereas M.D. students are typically trained to be clinicians. Perhaps more relevant to M.D. training in psychiatry, Ph.D. students in clinical psychology appear to be somewhat more successful at research career tracking than their counterparts who earn Psy.D. degrees. This is relevant because, although both Ph.D. and Psy.D. clinical psychologists are trained to treat patients, Ph.D. degree holders are more likely to have been schooled under the "Boulder method," which emphasizes the scientist-practitioner model. Under that model, psychology graduate students receive at least 3 years of training in research design, methodology, and psychological assessment, and they also are required to complete an independent dissertation involving the collection of empirical data (Belar and Perry, 1992). The consequence of that training may well be related to participation in clinical research by Ph.D. psychologists, as a 1988 survey of 250 Ph.D. and 137 Psy.D. recipients found that 7.4 percent of the Ph.D. degree holders identified themselves as "primarily researchers," whereas none of the Psy.D.'s did so (Barrom et al., 1988).

The reality that psychologists are more apt to conduct research is clearly demonstrated by the relative numbers of M.D. and Ph.D. degree holders who apply for federal grants, as well as by their comparative involvement in the formal grant application evaluation process. From 1987 to 2001, 60 to 70 percent of all National Institute of Mental Health (NIMH) grant awardees were Ph.D.'s, compared with the 30 to 40 percent who were M.D.'s or M.D./Ph.D.'s. (see Figure 5-2). It is notable, however, that success rates for Ph.D.s, M.D.'s, and M.D./Ph.D.'s are almost identical, averaging between 20 and 40 percent (see Figure 5-3). Other studies have presented similar findings (IOM, 2000; Nathan, 1998; Wyngaarden, 1979; Zemlo et al., 2000), suggesting strongly that while physicians are competitive for federal grants, they apply for such grants in far lower numbers than Ph.D.'s—a reality that in all probability impacts negatively on the number of patient-oriented research projects.

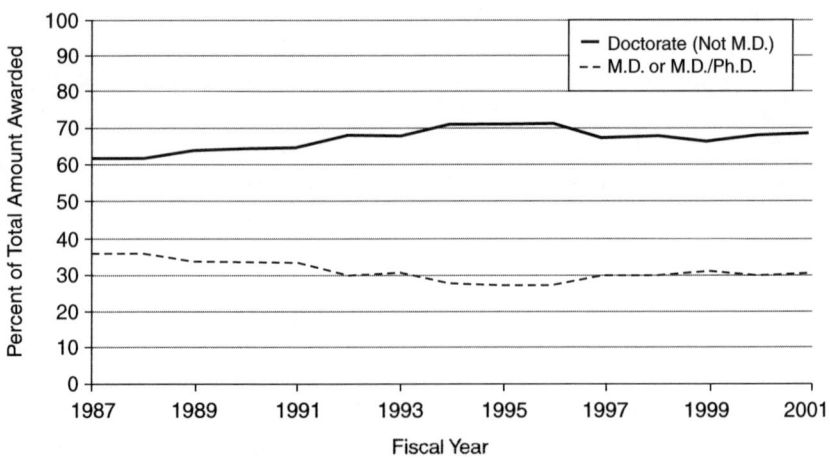

FIGURE 5-2 Percent of National Institute of Mental Health (NIMH) research project grants that were awarded to principal investigators, stratified by highest degree (e.g., M.D).
SOURCE: Plot courtesy of the NIMH, Office of Science Policy and Program Policy, February 21, 2003.

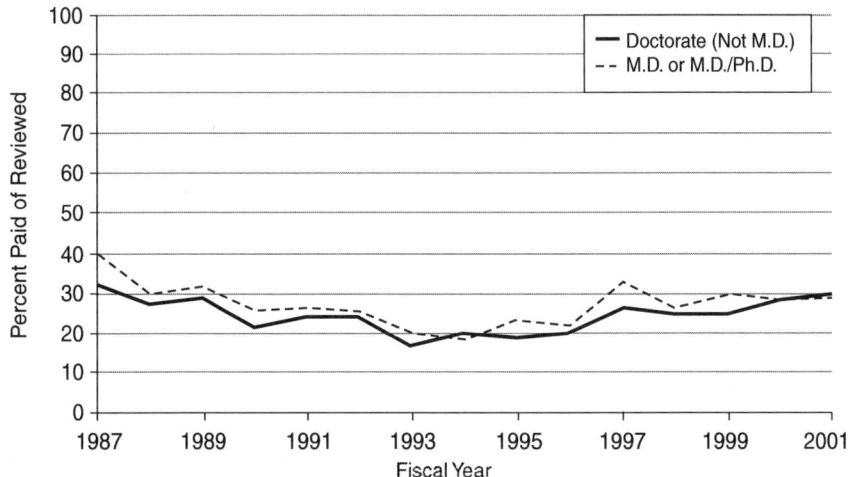

FIGURE 5-3 Success rate of National Institute of Mental Health (NIMH) research project grant applications, stratified by degree of the principal investigator. Success rate = number funded/number applied.
SOURCE: Plot courtesy of the NIMH, Office of Science Policy and Program Policy, February 21, 2003.

In addition to data indicating that M.D. applicants are competitive for federal research grants, the funding anxieties of trainees can be assuaged if they are educated about the training and career development grants that are available to help them develop research and grant preparation skills they may lack because they have not had Ph.D. training. The K-award is the most notable example of such training (see Chapter 2). Additionally, there are numerous masters degree and certificate programs available for residents, fellows, and junior faculty, especially for the latter two groups (as discussed in Chapter 2). Finally, there are local and national seminars and workshops that offer pragmatic information about the overall grant application process. For example, there is an annual 1.5-day NIMH Workshop on Child and Adolescent Research that is focused on providing participants with research career information, including study design, statistics, and "grantsmanship" issues (NIMH, 2002a). Similar local programs have been developed at leading research centers, such as Western Psychiatric Institute and Clinic (WPIC). Although these programs do not ensure success in obtaining grants, they may be helping. It was found that 16 of 30 (52 percent) second-year fellows at WPIC who had taken the "grantsmanship" seminar had received some extramural funding by the end of their fellowship (Reynolds et al., 1998)—a proportion that may represent an increase in extramural funding attainment since a 1989 survey indicated that academic psychiatrists typically did not obtained their first grant until 3 years after completing their research training (Pincus et al., 1995).

REPRESENTATION OF WOMEN, INTERNATIONAL MEDICAL GRADUATES, AND RACIAL MINORITIES IN PSYCHIATRY

Gender, country of origin, and race are three immutable personal characteristics that have an impact on career paths in psychiatry, including research careers. The principal aim of this section is to consider those characteristics in light of the need for training programs to foster productive research careers among the most diverse and talented workforce available. Table 5-4 summarizes the demographics of psychiatry and several other specialties of medicine in 1999. The table shows that psychiatry attracts a relatively high number of women, international medical graduates (IMGs), and underrepresented racial and ethnic minorities as compared with most other specialties of medicine. Psychiatry appears to attract more females than do most medical specialties. IMGs are overrepresented in psychiatry, accounting for 42.9 percent of residents, compared with 26.4 percent of residents across medicine. The table also shows that, while psychiatry does attract more minorities than many other medical specialties, the discipline falls well short of attracting a number that is proportional to the general U.S. minority population (11.7 percent versus 25.4 percent).

Data from the American Medical Association indicate that from 1970 to 1990, about 2 to 6 percent of all physicians, female physicians, and IMG physicians considered research their primary professional activity (Pasko and Seidman, 2002). Sometime between 1985 and 1990, however, a precipitous decline occurred whereby fewer than 3 percent of each of these three groups considered research their main activity, and research involvement by IMGs and women both dropped sharply and below that among all physicians (see Figure 5-4). One interpretation of this shift is that women and IMGs have been given greater clinical opportunities in recent years. It may be, however, that the special needs of IMGs and women are not being fully considered in the context of research training. Accordingly, the following sections detail research training issues faced by women, IMGs, and underrepresented racial and ethnic minority groups.

TABLE 5-4 Demographic Composition of Residents in Various Specialties or Subspecialties of Medicine, August 1999

Specialty	% Female (rank)	% International Medical Graduates[a] (rank)	% Underrepresented Minority[b] (rank)
Obstetrics-Gynecology	67.2 (1)	7.5 (8)	16.8 (1)
Pediatrics	64.6 (2)	19.5 (6)	13.8 (2)
Psychiatry	49.0 (3)	42.9 (3)	11.7 (3)
Pathology	46.9 (4)	48.5 (2)	7.0 (7)
Allergy and Immunology	44.0 (5)	42.1 (4)	6.7 (8)
Internal Medicine	39.6 (6)	37.2 (5)	10.7 (4)
Neurology	36.2 (7)	49.4 (1)	8.1 (6)
General Surgery	21.2 (8)	13.7 (7)	10.1 (5)
Orthopedic Surgery	7.8 (9)	2.0 (9)	6.1 (9)
Total Among Medical Residents[c]	38.1	26.4	10.7
Total in U.S. Population[d]	50.9	N/A	25.4

[a] International medical graduates are all physicians who received their undergraduate medical education in a non-U.S. medical school. This number does not include graduates of Canadian medical schools.
[b] Underrepresented minority is defined as Hispanic or African American.
[c] Total based on information for 28 specialties.
[d] U.S. census data for 2000.
SOURCE: Journal of the American Medical Association (2000); U.S. Bureau of the Census (2002).

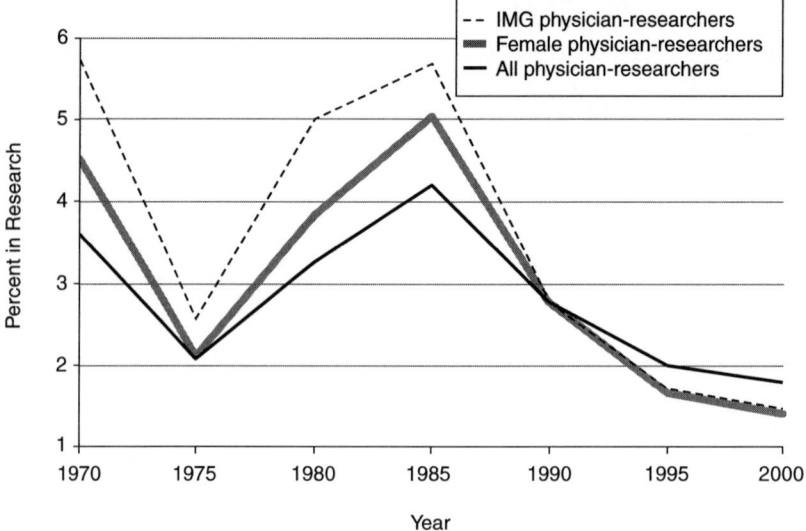

FIGURE 5-4 Total number (table) and percentages (graph) of all, female, and international medical graduate (IMG) physicians declaring research as their primary activity, 1970–2000.
SOURCE: Pasko and Seidman (2002).

Women

In 2001 and 2002, women accounted for nearly half of U.S. medical students and represented 51 percent of psychiatry residents, whereas in 1989 and 1990, they made up just 36 percent of medical students and 41 percent of psychiatry residents (Bickel et al., 2002a). These increasing numbers of women who are both medical students and psychiatry residents have implications for research training.

Unfortunately, the above increases do not translate into a large number of female physician-investigators in the field of psychiatry. In their study of the research involvement of psychiatrists, Haviland and colleagues note that "an increasing number of psychiatrists are women and there is evidence that fewer women than men go into research careers" (1987:80). Similarly, Leibenluft and colleagues (1993) conducted a survey of 1,923 full-time psychiatry department faculty members who had received their medical degree from 1956 to 1985, and found that for the years 1976 to 1985, nearly three-quarters of male psychiatrists in academic settings had conducted research, compared with about half of female psychiatrists. Furthermore, Leibenluft and colleagues (1993:896) found that "men were more likely than women to have had research training, to have ever been principal investigators on peer-reviewed grants, to mentor research trainees, [and] to be currently involved in research activities..." Specifically, more than 50 percent of men and only 40 percent of women had received research training in medical school; 30 percent of men had received postdoctoral research training, compared with 18 percent of women; and men were twice as likely as women to be principal investigators on peer-reviewed grants or to have mentored research trainees.

Some progress may have occurred since the above studies were conducted in the late 1980s. However, 2001 data from NIMH suggest that female researchers in psychiatry still fall well behind their male counterparts. Specifically, in fiscal year 2001 there were 574 male psychiatrists who were principal investigators on grants, compared with only 122 female investigators (i.e., 18 percent of psychiatrist-investigators were female). Other female M.D.'s were only slightly better represented within their discipline than psychiatrists (19 percent), but perhaps most revealing is the fact that for all other major categories of investigators (i.e., biological scientists, psychologists, and social scientists), involvement of females in the NIMH research pool ranged from 30 to 50 percent (data courtesy of NIMH, Office of Science Policy and Program Policy, February 21, 2003).

There are a number of reasons why female psychiatrists do not conduct research or do so to a lesser degree than male psychiatrists. First, female psychiatrists may have chosen their field because it provides both flexibility and the opportunity to balance career and family obligations. These interests can be compromised by the time demands of sustaining a credible research agenda, despite the fact that academic pursuits do offer some relief from the constraints of full-time clinical work, as mentioned earlier in this chapter. Indeed, many female physicians work part-time or take extended leave to have children (Cull et al., 2002; Culliton, 1984;

McMurray et al., 2002). Roeske (1976) found that female psychiatrists tend to have interrupted their training to have children, are more likely to have alternative working arrangements (part-time) than men, and work 30 percent fewer hours than men. A more recent survey of nearly 600 female psychiatrists and 4,000 other female physicians by Frank et al. (2001a) found that female psychiatrists work fewer hours than other female physicians, with age-adjusted mean hours worked being 38.5 and 43.9, respectively.

Second, those who work part-time or take extended leave may be at a disadvantage in academia, where publications and continual research funding are key factors in obtaining tenure. A report by Leibenluft et al. (1993:903) noted that "small differences in productivity between junior scientists tend to enlarge over time, as those who are more productive accrue resources that allow their scientific output to grow exponentially in the ensuing years." Although some academic institutions have begun to recognize this disadvantage and delay tenure decisions for women or male primary caretakers, many have not (Andrews, 2002).

Third, female psychiatry residents may be less likely to pursue research tracks than men because there are few women role models or mentors to inspire them in this direction (Leibenluft et al., 1993; Osborn et al., 1992). A recent report by Bickel et al. of the AAMC (2002b) notes that few medical schools have a critical mass of women leaders who can be inspiring role models to female physicians. Indeed, in 2002, only 37 percent of psychiatry faculty members were women (Bickel et al., 2002a). It is reasonable to expect that the percentage of female faculty members who conduct research is even more marginal.

International Medical Graduates

IMGs are U.S. citizens and non-U.S. citizens who graduated from a non-U.S. or non-Canadian medical school. Like women, IMGs make up a substantial proportion of psychiatry residents. Specifically, although IMGs account for slightly more than one-quarter of all U.S. medical residents (see Table 5-4), they account for more than 40 percent of psychiatry residents (Balon et al., 1999; Brotherton et al., 2002; Council of Graduate Medical Education [COGME], 1998; Mullan, 2000). Figure 5-5 summarizes data for 1992 to 2002 from the National Resident Matching Program (NRMP) on the numbers of foreign- and U.S.-born IMGs and the numbers of U.S. medical school graduates entering psychiatry as first-year postgraduate (PGY1) residents.

Figure 5-5 indicates that the number of foreign IMGs peaked in 1997 (34 percent of all PGY1 residents) and has gradually declined since that time. That decline has been offset slightly by an increase in the number of U.S. citizen IMGs and U.S. senior medical students entering psychiatry residency programs. This suggests that general recruitment to the field has improved since many institutions favor U.S. medical school graduates as candidates for their residency programs.

For U.S. IMGs, the path to residency and research training is similar to that for U.S. medical school graduates. However, foreign IMGs face at least three obstacles en route to postgraduate medical research training. First, along with the USMLE, they must pass a clinical skills assessment (e.g., history taking, physical exams, communicating with patients in spoken English) to be certified for U.S. medical residency programs (Whelan et al., 2002). Second, foreign physicians are required to obtain appropriate visas (e.g., J-1) to enter and study in this country, and are

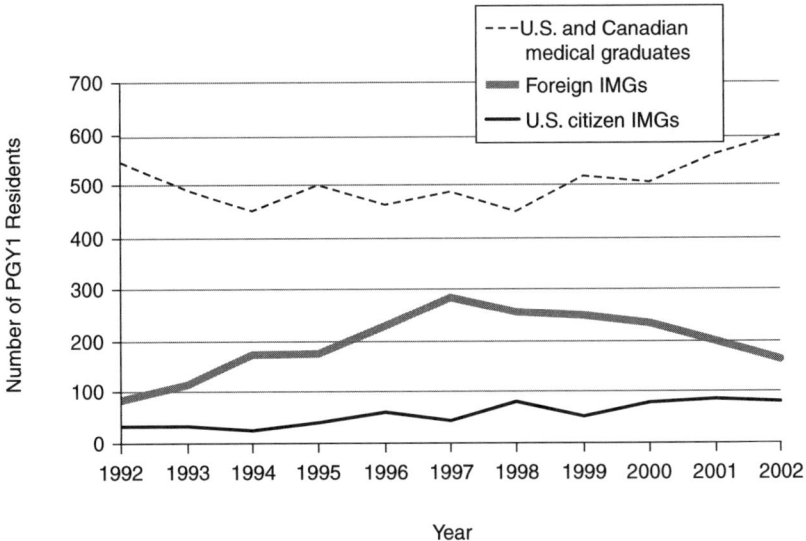

FIGURE 5-5 Number of international medical graduates (IMGs) (both foreign and U.S. citizens who graduated from foreign medical schools) and U.S. medical graduates (including Canadian graduates) who entered psychiatry as PGY1 residents. International medical graduates are those who attended a non-U.S. medical school.
SOURCE: Data from the National Resident Matching Program Data Warehouse, 1992–2002 (as of March 27, 2003).

then required to return to their country for 2 years before applying for permanent status in the United States (Baer et al., 1998) unless they agree to serve in areas with unmet health professional needs (Baer et al., 1999). Third, IMGs on temporary or student visas are ineligible for grants such as National Research Service Award fellowships and training grants and mentored career awards (NIH, 2000a; 2002b; 2003c). The result is that talented and ambitious IMGs may be prevented from enrolling in research training programs. This situation may contribute to a substantial loss in the number of patient-oriented researchers not only in this country, but also in other countries to which these individuals might potentially contribute should they decide to return home or emigrate elsewhere.

The committee agrees with the utility of screening non-U.S. medical graduates for basic skills; once these requirements have been met, however, outstanding residents should be given full opportunities to engage in research training and to contribute to psychiatric research, as many foreign IMGs have made important contributions in the past (Balon et al., 1999). Akin to allowing IMGs to serve in geographic areas with a need for health professionals, Congress should consider designating specific areas of research training and patient-oriented research activities as federally underserved *disciplines*, thereby permitting individuals who have demonstrated the necessary aptitude and ambition to train as patient-oriented researchers. The committee is fully aware that the current political climate makes such a suggestion controversial, but believes it to be appropriate given the previous success experienced by psychiatry and other fields of medicine with IMG researchers and the need for more physicians to be engaged in patient-oriented research.

Underrepresented Racial and Ethnic Minorities

Unlike women and IMGs, certain racial and ethnic minorities, including African Americans, Hispanics, and Native Americans, represent a limited proportion of psychiatrists in general and investigators in particular. As noted in Table 5-4, in 1999 African Americans and Hispanics composed just over one-quarter of the U.S. population and just over 11 percent of psychiatric residents. In that same year, however, fewer than 6 percent of all applicants for NIMH funding and fewer than 4 percent of all applicants receiving such funding came from those minorities (National Advisory Mental Health Council's Workgroup on Racial/Ethnic Diversity in Research Training and Health Disparities Research, 2001).

Minorities may not engage in research activity for at least two reasons. First, minorities, and particularly African Americans, tend to be suspicious of the mental health system, as they are at increased risk of being misdiagnosed, committed or incarcerated, or inappropriately medicated (DHHS, 2001a; IOM, 2003; Lawson, 1996; 2000). Second, as with women, there is also a shortage of ethnic and racial minorities who can serve as research role models for medical students. Data indicate that African Americans, Hispanics, and Native Americans are underrepresented as full-time faculty in health science, natural science, and social science departments (National Advisory Mental Health Council's Workgroup on Racial/Ethnic Diversity in Research Training and Health Disparities Research, 2001). Data from 2001 indicate that fewer than 5 percent of full-time medical faculty with an M.D. are underrepresented minorities (The Robert Wood Johnson Foundation, 2003). During most of the 1990s, there was only one African American psychiatrist with a career development award or an R01 grant, and that number has since increased only marginally.[36] Additionally, African American students are disproportionately trained at historically black colleges and universities, which before 2001 received no federal funding for psychiatrists (National Advisory Mental Health Council's Workgroup on Racial/Ethnic Diversity in Research Training and Health Disparities Research, 2001). Given that almost 29 percent of African American medical school graduates attended such colleges and universities from 1950 to 1998 (IOM, 2001b), it is imperative that these institutions develop and promote their research infrastructure to ensure an adequate supply of minority mental health researchers who can serve as role models. As noted during a recent workshop on minority training hosted by NIMH:

> With a lack of networking/mentoring comes a lack of advice, of acknowledgment, considerations for positions, publications and funding. Additionally, appropriate mentors are needed who understand and can help students make the language 'shift' from their heritage and culture to the 'mainstream.' (NIMH, 1999: 7)

Although racial and ethnic minorities face a number of obstacles in becoming researchers, there are also numerous opportunities for members of these groups to receive research training support. However, these opportunities appear to be insufficient to attract large numbers of appli-

---

[36]Based on the committee's review of the Computer Retrieval of Information on Scientific Projects (CRISP) database.

cants. Research training grants and fellowships often target minorities. Additionally, the National Institutes of Health (NIH) funds minority supplement grants to encourage senior investigators to mentor minority trainees in the context of their ongoing work (National Advisory Mental Health Council's Workgroup on Racial/Ethnic Diversity in Research Training and Health Disparities Research, 2001). Success rates among applicants for such grants are very high: of 51 applications for NIMH minority supplement grants submitted in 1998, 100 percent were funded, for a combined total of almost $5.5 million (NIMH, 2000a). Several professional societies in psychiatry also offer research training opportunities for minorities. Other minority funding opportunities include an NIMH-supported T32 grant first received by the APA in 1989 to develop a program aimed at minority research training in psychiatry (see Chapter 2). The American Academy of Child and Adolescent Psychiatry also has funding programs targeting scholarships and fellowships for minorities (see Appendix B for additional information on funding opportunities).

Recognizing the need for mentor support, a recent NIMH report recommends the creation of a national mentoring network of senior minority and nonminority investigators to develop extended relationships with minority trainees and investigators (National Advisory Mental Health Council's Workgroup on Racial/Ethnic Diversity in Research Training and Health Disparities Research, 2001). Mentoring for minorities has already been addressed directly at some universities. For example, a 1998 review of the mentoring program of the University of Pennsylvania found that minority physicians were unsuccessful at finding research mentors, and those minority physicians who were mentors were overburdened with the additional responsibilities of serving on committees and task forces to ensure minority representation (Johnson et al., 1998). To remedy the situation, the university aggressively recruited minority faculty such that between 1993 and 1997, their numbers increased by 32 percent. This hiring effort was coupled with general counseling, research development, training in research methods, and grant writing (Johnson et al., 1998). Similarly, to increase the number of minority faculty, Harvard University created the Minority Faculty Development Program in 1991 to encourage medical students to consider careers in academia and to promote career development of junior faculty (Curry, 1997; Potts, 1992). Yet another important example of strategies to build a critical mass of minority researchers is NIMH's use of the R24 mechanism to award Minority Research Infrastructure Support Program (M-RISP) grants to a number of institutions to support mental health research and individual investigator/faculty development. The M-RISP is awarded to institutions with a significant number (greater than 30 percent) of racial and ethnic minority students or to a Native American tribe that applies in collaboration with a mental health training institution. Awards are made for 3 to 5 years, depending on whether the grant application is new or renewable, at a maximum direct cost of $400,000 (NIH, 2000c).

Thus it is apparent that there is considerable funding for minority researchers. However, many of those targeted by these opportunities either are not aware of the funding or lack the core resources that would allow them to prepare an application. Outreach efforts to educate minority psychiatrists about these grants would likely increase those applications. Furthermore, it is important that fledgling researchers receive guidance and mentoring from senior psychiatrist-researchers to ensure adequate recruitment and retention.

CONCLUSIONS AND RECOMMENDATIONS

Individuals considering patient-oriented research in psychiatry are likely influenced by a number of personal factors. Some of these factors are so intrinsic that it is difficult to imagine the formal educational process, especially in adulthood, having much impact on them. For example, perhaps the best any discipline can do with regard to candidates having exceptional drive or talent is to encourage them toward that specialty. There is some evidence that psychiatry may not be competitive in attracting the top medical students, despite unparalleled opportunities in the clinical brain and behavioral sciences. Part of the problem may be the compensation of psychiatrists as compared with that for other disciplines. The anticipated salaries for psychiatrists, whether academic or practicing, are near the bottom of the physician pay scale. Accordingly, concerns about loan repayment and overall financial well-being may discourage potential patient-oriented researchers from extended research training that would further delay them from achieving their full earning potential. Accordingly, one obvious recommendation the committee makes is as follows:

> **Recommendation 5.1. The National Institute of Mental Health and other funding agencies should seek mechanisms to offer increased financial incentives, such as loan repayment, to trainees who commit to research training and research involvement beyond core psychiatry residency.**

The committee encourages these agencies to be creative in designing ways to increase or otherwise supplement training stipends for promising psychiatry trainees. Maintaining and expanding loan repayment programs will likely be an important part of this strategy. As early as 1989, NIH offered debt-repayment grants to physician-researchers. NIH intramural and extramural debt-relief grants have included those targeting certain diseases (e.g., HIV, infertility), patient populations (e.g., children, minorities), and clinical research specifically (IOM, 1994; Ley and Rosenberg, 2002; Nathan, 2002; NIH, 2002a). In 2002, NIMH budgeted $2.5 million for its loan repayment program to support 53 trainees and junior faculty. Recipients receive a maximum of $35,000 each year for up to 2 years, during which time they commit to at least 20 research hours each week. The budget was doubled for 2003, and eligibility was expanded to include those who do not have an NIH grant. In 2002, 82 percent of all applicants to the NIMH program were funded, this high rate likely being due to the fact that the program was new and thus not broadly known among potential applicants (NIMH, 2002d). What remains to be seen is whether these grants will entice more individuals to become researchers or simply reward those already on the research track (Pardes, 2002).

Despite the absence of direct evidence, it is axiomatic that debt relief will attract some young psychiatrists to research, and survey data support this hypothesis. For example, a recent web-based survey of 86 neurology residents found that loan repayment incentives would encourage 76 percent of those residents to consider extended postresidency research training that included "the expectation of future practice in academic neurology" (Doherty et al., 2002). Given that 63 percent of this sample intended to become academics, it is most important that 15 of 17 individuals who expressed uncertainty about an academic career and 8 of 15 who had previously ruled out such a path responded favorably to the idea of research training if it were supported with loan repayment assistance. Loan repayment programs are likely to be attractive to trainees with considerable debt, particularly members of underrepresented minorities, who typically graduate with higher levels of debt than students overall (NIMH, 1999; National Research Council [NRC], 2000; Spar et al., 1993). Furthermore, the Surgeon General's report on mental health notes that African Americans have only one-tenth the net worth of Caucasians (DHHS, 2001a).

A complementary strategy to loan repayment is for funding agencies to supplement research training stipends as they are well below the income levels one could expect from direct entry into clinical practice. In 2003, for example, the annual stipend for someone in their fifth year of training after medical school was just over $44,000 (NIH, 2003d), well below the entry level salary of a junior psychiatrists which are double or triple that amount (see Table 5-2). Accordingly, the committee believes that increasing compensation represents an important and obvious way to encourage more residents to undertake additional training before entering their first full-paying position.

Stipend amounts for training are determined largely under the authority of the Secretary of Health and Human Services. The remuneration is designed principally to defray living expenses incurred during training, and thus federal legislation dating back to 1974 requires M.D. and Ph.D. fellows to receive the same stipend levels (NRC, 2000). This structuring means that stipend increases for psychiatrists or even physician-investigators in isolation are not likely under the current system.

Provisions for supplementing income, via moonlighting or non-federal sources, however is permitted by NIH regulations (NIH, 2001a). Columbia University, for example, has several fellowship programs, and the state provides funding to increase training stipends (Rieder, 2001; 2003). The department of neurology at the University of Rochester also permits research fellows to negotiate their compensation arrangements based on their productivity in applying for extramural funding (Griggs, 2002). Alternatively, some institutions allow research training to overlap with junior faculty status as an incentive to potential researchers. Foundations, philanthropists, and other third-party supporters also represent important potential sources of funding for financial incentives to trainees committed to patient-oriented research careers.

In the case of residents, whose time is limited by the demands of clinical training, department funds might be used to increase residency compensation by creating "research moonlighting" opportunities, a practice currently in place at Columbia University (personal communication, R. Rieder, Columbia University, April 2003). At Columbia, research moonlighting typically engages one resident per year and involves chart review or some other research activity that can be carried out on a part-time basis. To the extent that such arrangements lead to a meaningful product and give residents hands-on experience, they may serve the dual purpose of training and of supplementing personal income.

Ultimately, recommendation 5.1 is about investing in the trainee specifically—not to make training compensation equal to the pay one would receive as an independent practitioner or investigator, but to increase the probability that a few more young psychiatrists will prolong their full-time educational experience to pursue the goal of developing into an independent patient-oriented researcher.

Although financial expectations play a role in their career decisions, medical students and residents are equally if not more concerned about other issues, such as lifestyle and the intellectual content of their selected profession. Furthermore, new physicians are understandably anxious about the challenges involved in securing long-term research funding. The committee observed that in recent years, several well-respected editorial writers have written extensively about the problems associated with clinical research without promoting the endeavor as an exciting option for new physicians (Lieberman, 2001; Schrier, 1997; Shine, 1998). The preface to a recent opinion piece by an established psychiatrist-researcher, for example, notes that research careers are not glamorous, may not be intellectually exciting, are tedious, and typically involve considerable delayed gratification (Lieberman, 2001). While such characterizations are partially true of most hard-earned achievements, the committee is concerned that they may inappropriately overshadow the positive aspects of a research career. Thus we make the following recommendation:

> **Recommendation 5.2. Individuals and institutions involved in the education and mentoring of medical students, residents and fellows should strongly convey to these trainees the benefits (professional and societal) associated with patient-oriented research in psychiatry. Promotion strategies might include support for student interest groups; brochures, websites, and other media; and summer research training opportunities.**

This recommendation is based on two principles: first, research offers a number of nonsalary benefits that can at least partially offset the demands and financial concerns associated with a research career (see Box 5-1 above); second, stakeholders should promote these benefits at all stages of training (i.e., during undergraduate education, medical school, residency, and fellowship). As discussed in Chapter 2, early exposure to research opportunities is one of the few correlates to a sustained research career. The above recommendation is made to encourage recruitment strategies that emphasize the growing scientific evidence base underlying the practice of modern psychiatry (Charney et al., 2001; Goldman, 2002). As obvious as this recommendation may appear, the committee nevertheless believes such promotion strategies are logically and plainly tied to recruiting students and residents to research careers. The committee furthermore believes that the typical dialogue regarding research in general and clinical research in particular focuses so much on problems that it is no wonder that many medical students shy away from the endeavor. Implementation of this recommendation should not involve a concealment of the challenges to patient-oriented research (e.g., standardization of complex treatments and symptoms, struggles for funding), but instead should strive to present the positives along side the negatives.

Finally, the demographics of the psychiatry workforce suggest that special measures are needed to ensure that talented women and IMGs are encouraged to pursue careers in patient-oriented research. Additionally, as is the case for all branches of medicine, greater involvement of underrepresented minorities is imperative if psychiatry is to offer the most responsive care to a diverse U.S. population. Accordingly, the committee makes the three recommendations presented below.

> **Recommendation 5.3. Departments of psychiatry, supported by the National Institute of Mental Health and other psychiatric organizations, should provide leadership in recruiting and retaining more women for psychiatry research careers. Such efforts should include:**
>
> - **Increasing part-time training and job sharing opportunities.**
> - **Developing a critical mass of female role models and mentors.**
> - **Working with institutions to improve child day care programs.**
> - **Addressing institutional promotion and tenure issues, such as the tenure clock, that may be perceived as barriers to female trainees.**
> - **Educating women about the time flexibility of research careers.**

Considerable progress has already been made in this area, so there are numerous programmatic examples from which to draw. A 1996 report published by the AAMC outlines some programs that provide a supportive infrastructure for female trainees and faculty members across medicine. Some of these programs offer mentoring support (e.g., Loma Linda University), provide child care (e.g., Beth Israel Hospital in Boston), and support part-time opportunities and flexible scheduling (e.g. University of Virginia), while others track faculty development and review promotion and salary policies to ensure that the needs of women faculty and trainees are considered (e.g., University of California at Davis, Stanford University, Johns Hopkins University, Harvard University) (AAMC, 1996).

> **Recommendation 5.4. Psychiatry training programs, academic medical centers, psychiatry organizations, and the federal government should work together to facilitate research training for international medical graduates who have the potential to make outstanding research contributions to psychiatry. Retention of the most productive of these international graduates in U.S. academic psychiatry programs should also be a joint effort.**

The committee is not aware of any institutions or psychiatry residency training programs that focus on accommodating the unique needs of IMGs. However, certain professional organizations have addressed some of the issues faced by these individuals. For example, the American Association of Directors of Psychiatric Residency Training has established a mentoring program for IMG residents (AADPRT, 2003). The APA, with funding from the Pfizer Company, publishes *The International Psychiatrist Newsletter*, which offers support and information to IMGs in psychiatry (APA, 1997b). Finally, a possible model for training foreign IMGs may come from the Epidemic Intelligence Service, which offers classroom- and field-based training to 60 to 80 health professionals, including 8 to 10 foreign trainees, each year (Centers for Disease Control and Prevention, 2002; White et al., 2001). Similar programs that increase international cooperation in the area of mental health research might enhance not only psychiatric research efforts in the United States, but also mental health efforts internationally. The committee believes recommendation 5.4 is especially important given the new visa restrictions faced by non-U.S. IMGs in the wake of the 2001 terrorist attacks.

> **Recommendation 5.5. Psychiatry research training programs should increase the numbers of underrepresented minority researchers by employing the following strategies:**

- **Recruit minority faculty in multiple disciplines to serve as role models and mentors.**
- **Pursue funding from NIMH and other funding agencies that support minority trainees and faculty.**
- **Inform more minority psychiatrists about research training and other funding opportunities.**

Data indicate that racial and ethnic minorities apply in relatively low numbers for NIMH funds (National Advisory Mental Health Council's Workgroup on Racial/Ethnic Diversity in Research Training and Health Disparities Research, 2001). One option for reversing this trend is to make minority medical students and psychiatrists more aware of the opportunities and needs that exist in patient-oriented research (Curry, 1997). Low application rates may, in no small part, be related to the fact that minority medical students often are from families with limited accumulated wealth, and thus they become highly dependent on loans or are otherwise constrained from career paths that delay full financial remuneration. Therefore, increased stipends and loan repayment programs (per recommendation 5.1) may be of particular relevance to minorities. Structured programs to match minorities to role models with similar experiences and to build a minority presence in departments have been engineered at some institutions (e.g., University of Pennsylvania), and these programs represent examples for others to emulate.

6

Future Directions for Promoting the Development of Psychiatrist-Researchers

This report has described the importance of early research training for the development of independent patient-oriented researchers in psychiatry. It has also reviewed regulatory, institutional, and personal factors that are relevant to such training. This final chapter addresses three overarching issues that the committee believes are important for the future of psychiatric research training. The first is the importance of having better and more data regarding the research workforce and society's need for psychiatrist-researchers. The second is the need for more outcome data in ongoing and novel patient-oriented research training efforts. These outcome data should describe, at a minimum, the frequency with which a given strategy yields a bona fide researcher. Third is the need for a national effort to promote, implement, and monitor the training of psychiatrist-researchers. To be effective at recruiting researchers and raising financial support for the costs of training, such an effort should be directed at medical students and residents on the one hand and society at large on the other. The chapter ends with an overarching recommendation addressing these needs.

WORKFORCE ESTIMATES AND MONITORING

As discussed in Chapter 1, the committee had considerable difficulty finding data regarding the current size of the psychiatrist-researcher workforce, as well as projected needs. Although it is clear that psychiatrist-researchers have made and continue to make contributions to patient-oriented investigations, it is not clear how many psychiatrist-researchers need to be trained to replace those who are retiring or otherwise leaving the workforce. It is also not known how many additional psychiatrist-researchers are needed given the increasing importance of mental health to the nation's overall health. Part of the problem is in establishing a precise definition of a psychiatrist-researcher. Is a psychiatrist-researcher someone who does research 1 day a week (Pincus et al., 1995), or must research be the primary professional activity (AAMC, 2002b)? Are psychiatrist-researchers those who serve as principal investigators on federal research grants, or is it sufficient for them to serve as consultants on late-phase clinical trials? In *The Crisis in Clinical Research*, Ahrens (1992) argues that the latter type of research (e.g., trials of emerging drugs and devices) will readily attract capital resources, and thus particular attention should be directed to more innovative types of research that will expand our knowledge of the disease process in more complex ways. In any case, characterization of the current and desired psychiatrist-research workforce is essential to determine who should be trained and in what methods.

Determining the future need for researchers is more difficult than determining the numbers and types of current researchers. Workforce needs estimates in medicine are generally difficult to calculate. Measuring the physician workforce with regard to the projected needs of various specialties is extremely difficult, if not impossible, to do with great precision (Council of Graduate Medical Education [COGME], 2000). As recently as 1996, a serious oversupply of physicians was predicted (Knapp, 2002), but by June 2002, the Association of American Medical Colleges (AAMC) had released the following policy statement:

> After reviewing the range of studies over the past several decades…the AAMC has concluded that no definitive conclusion can be drawn about the adequacy of the workforce, nor can specific recommendations be made about the rate of supply of new physicians (Knapp, 2002:1078).

A recent National Research Council (NRC) report on the training of junior biomedical and behavioral scientists calls for increasing the numbers of physician-researchers based on a relative decline in those numbers and on the following logic:

> Because those who interact with patients often bring great understanding and awareness of the health needs of the public to clinical research, the diminishing role played by physicians affects the capacity of the clinical research workforce to sustain a program of research that addresses the nation's needs (NRC, 2000:51).

As sound as that logic may appear, it would be strengthened by studies quantitatively demonstrating the public health impact of patient-oriented physician-investigators. As described in Chapter 1, the great burden of mental illness and the unique skills of psychiatrists together allow one to conclude that a low number of psychiatrist-researchers is detrimental to the nation's overall ability to cope with mental illness. However, this is indirect evidence at best, and thus the committee believes it will be important for psychiatry to demonstrate more directly the importance of training greater numbers of researchers to justify the resources necessary for that training. The committee had difficulty identifying published studies that explicitly quantify the benefits associated with research conducted by psychiatrists. However, we found one study that demonstrated impressive cost savings associated with psychiatric research more generally (Silverstein et al., 1995). Additionally, the committee performed two rudimentary assessments of recent publications first-authored by psychiatrists, and job listings in psychiatric research, both of which indicated the importance of or demand for psychiatrist-initiated research. These types of reviews offer models for more thorough investigations in the future (see Box 6-1 for details).

An alternative hypothesis to the idea that there is an increasing gap between mental health needs and the number of psychiatrist-researchers is that there is instead, or additionally, a shortage of other professionals in mental health and mental health research (e.g., clinicians, psychologists, social workers, neuropharmacologists). Although such workforce estimates are beyond the committee's charge of identifying strategies to increase the numbers of psychiatrists engaged in research, the committee believes sound workforce estimates are necessary for planning and implementing a credible training effort. At least one recent study takes a national look at the composition of the clinical mental health workforce and finds that while the numbers of psychiatrists in that workforce have increased markedly (by 15 percent) since the early 1990s, the numbers of psychologists and social workers have increased at even higher rates (37 percent and 18 percent, respectively) (Scheffler and Kirby, 2003). Similar trends are implied by studies of physician-investigators and Ph.D.-

investigators seeking support from the federal government (Zemlo et al., 2000). It is not well known, however, how psychiatrist-researchers have fared in recent years, and to what extent psychologists and other non-physician mental health practitioners have successfully filled the associated gaps in psychiatric patient-oriented research.

The Council on Research of the American Psychiatric Association (APA) has established the concrete goal of doubling the number of psychiatrist-researchers by 2012. However, that goal is based largely on impressions of leaders in the field, including those at the National Institute of Mental Health (NIMH), and on the broader decline in the numbers of all physician-investigators (personal communication, J. Greden, APA Council on Research, July 26, 2002). As the goal is based on neither a precise estimate of need nor trends specific to psychiatry, its importance may not be credible to decision makers outside of psychiatry.

BOX 6-1
**Three Studies Suggesting
the Need for Psychiatrist-Researchers**

Analysis of cost-savings. Silverstein and colleagues recently gathered cost-savings data from 19 medical and dental studies and found that biomedical innovations of the last 50 years have yielded approximately $69 billion in overall savings per year. They also found that nearly half of those savings ($33 billion per year) were the result of enhanced pharmacological therapies for patients suffering from schizophrenia or manic-depressive illness (Rosenberg, 2002; Silverstein et al., 1995).

Direct assessment of psychiatrist-initiated scholarship. In 2001, NIMH established a bibliography of brain and behavioral research studies for a White House Conference on mental health (NIMH, 2001b). A review of a randomly-selected subset (62 of 249) of first authors from that bibliography found that 50 percent were psychiatrists. The same bibliography of 249 citations was further reviewed by 13 lay reviewers with no connection to professional mental health practice and no knowledge of the aim of this IOM report. These lay reviewers were asked to peruse the bibliography and select articles they viewed as most important to the future of public mental health. More than half of these reviewers identified 10 articles as "important" and "compelling," and 6 of these were first-authored by psychiatrists. This informal assessment demonstrates that psychiatrists have a substantive presence as lead scholars on projects considered valuable to NIMH and the broader public as well.

Survey of the job market. Selected web-based issues of *Science* and of *Academic Physician and Scientist* were reviewed for faculty research position advertisements. The review took place on five separate days between late November and mid-December 2002, and late May and early June 2003. Web searches within each journal's job postings were done using the keywords corresponding to selected specialties (e.g., "psychiatry," "internal medicine"). Each position announcement was read to see whether research activity was part of the professional responsibilities involved and whether an M.D.-equivalent status was required. This review found 119 physician-researcher positions that translated into the following numbers per 10,000 practitioners in each field: psychiatry, 4.3 (n = 20); pediatrics, 3.9 (n = 25); internal medicine, 3.5* (n = 66); and neurology, 6.7 (n = 8). There are at least two important limitations to this survey. First, the sample size is very small, in part because the sample time was short. Second, it is improbable that the review assesses all or even the major sources of job openings for physician-researchers. A better assessment would involve polling department heads and reviewing specific trade journals and periodicals (e.g. for psychiatry, *Archives of General Psychiatry* or *Psychiatric News*). Nevertheless, the implication of this limited survey is that the demand for psychiatrist-researchers is at least as strong as that demand in other medical specialties, with the possible exception of neurology, another discipline focused on the clinical neurosciences, but one that is only one-quarter the size of the psychiatric workforce.

*Internal medicine in this survey included general internal medicine, cardiology, gastroenterology, geriatric medicine, hematology, infectious disease, nephrology, oncology, pulmonology, and rheumatology.

OUTCOME DATA IN RESEARCH TRAINING

The committee also experienced difficulty in obtaining outcome data regarding the success of national and local programs at training productive researchers. Outcome research in medical education is lacking at even the largest of medical institutions. A recent report of the Commonwealth Fund Taskforce on Academic Health Centers (2002) concludes that even at academic health centers, there is a lack of outcome data on effective education methods for training medical students and residents. Some programs (e.g., K23, K30; see Chapter 4) are admittedly too new to provide meaningful outcome data. However, it is the committee's strong impression that most programs do very little follow-up on residency or fellowship graduates to assess their professional activities. Although institutions and programs often make some estimate of how many researchers emerged from their educational efforts, the majority do not appear to differentiate between academic educators and academic researchers or between patient-oriented and basic researchers. Consequently, it is unclear what constitutes a "successful" research training program. Indeed, an informal outreach to training programs yielded a variety of different indices of success with regard to research training (see Chapter 4 and Appendix C for further details).

A standardized framework for assessing training programs is therefore needed to provide data on which strategies/programs are effective and which are not. Goldman and Williams (2001) have created a generic framework that could be applied to training inputs and outputs on a national and local basis. This framework is designed to help NIH with its data collection efforts and to "identify a range of possible policies and possible impact" of biomedical research (Goldman and Williams, 2001:4). This particular framework is offered as an example, not as an endorsement of its utility compared to other existing techniques for program evaluation.

Whatever framework is used, the committee believes strongly that qualitative and quantitative indices of research output by those who receive training or grant support should be periodically assessed to validate the effectiveness and impact of these programs and to consider ways to improve such research support mechanisms. The March of Dimes Birth Defect Foundation recently published an ambitious evaluation of their "Starter Scholar Research Award" grant program (Mavis and Katz, 2003). The evaluation reviewed the 10-year post-application, research productivity of 250 successful and 195 rejected applicants from the mid-1980s. Grant recipients were more prolific than non-recipients in terms of the number federal grant awards received and the number of publications produced. Additionally, awardee publications were cited twice as often as those from non-awardees (119 citations per paper per year, versus 48). Given that 84 percent of these awardees received at least one federal research grant, this study indicates that the March of Dimes has been quite successful at selecting applicants with future research potential. The study also found that successful applicants were more likely to be from prestigious institutions. Like many reports of this nature, however, this study does not offer any analyses that could be used to infer how the program might be expanded or improved to attract or train greater numbers of, and more productive, awardees.

Data on research training obtained by the committee typically focused on individual-trainee success stories with less frequent mention of those who failed to develop into researchers. These latter individuals arguably represent the most important group for follow-up study as they are a logical source of information regarding barriers to more efficient research training. It is obvious to the committee that such data are lacking for at least two reasons. First, success is difficult to define, since the quality of research is not necessarily captured by readily available indices, such as federal funding success or a tally of publications. Second, it is a potentially sensitive matter to contact individuals and programs regarding their "failures." A strong indication of this point comes from the March of Dimes review described above. As part of their assessment, Mavis and Katz (2003) sent a self-administered survey to all identified applicants. Responses to that survey came from 77 percent of the applicants who had succeeded at securing funding, but from only 28 percent of those who had failed. The failed applicants appear to have been far more reticent about their professional activities, perhaps because they were embarrassed or because they did not believe the survey to be valuable for their particular career objective. Whatever the case, to the extent that funders and association policy analysts want to identify ways of increasing the quality and quantity of grant applicants, they need to conduct evaluations that provide both endogenous (e.g., trainee opinions) and exogenous (e.g., grant priority scores, supervisor evaluations, online databases) information regarding former research trainees in at least three groups: (1) those who fail to achieve initial success, (2) those who opt out of research careers after early success, and (3) those who succeed and fail in categories of importance to the funder (e.g., patient-oriented research).

NATIONAL COORDINATING EFFORT

As described throughout this report, but especially in Chapters 3 and 4, the committee found that there are currently many professional societies and other stakeholders in mental health and psychiatry that are interested in and/or developing strategies to enhance patient-oriented research training for psychiatrists. As mentioned in Chapter 3, the American Academy of Child and Adolescent Psychiatry has a task force that has already drafted a research-oriented residency training schedule. The American Board of Psychiatry and Neurology (ABPN) and the Psychiatry Residency Review Committee (RRC) have been involved in such efforts, and leaders and members from those regulatory bodies appear to be interested in advancing research training during psychiatric training. Individual chairs and division heads also appear to believe unanimously that research training in psychiatry is important. The debate rests in how to make time and provide resources for implementing such activities given the demands and costs of clinical training and certification.

OVERARCHING RECOMMENDATION

Combining the apparent consensus on the importance of research training for psychiatrists with the conclusion that workforce estimates and outcome data are limited, the committee makes this final overarching recommendation:

> **Recommendation 6.1. The National Institute of Mental Health should take the lead in organizing a national body, including major stakeholders (e.g., patient groups, department chairs) and representatives of organizations in psychiatry, that will foster the integration of research into psychiatric residency and monitor outcomes of efforts to do so. This group should specifically collect and analyze relevant data, develop strategies to be put into practice, and measure the effectiveness of existing and novel approaches aimed at training patient-oriented researchers in psychiatry. The group should have direct consultative authority with the director of the National Institute of Mental Health, and also should provide concise periodic reports to all interested stakeholders regarding its accomplishments and future goals.**

NIMH should take the lead in implementing this recommendation by providing coordinated oversight of efforts to create a regular (e.g., annual) forum that convenes those interested in psychiatric research; furnishing financial resources for this forum to collect workforce and outcome data; and funding pilot initiatives to test potential training solutions. The seeds of such a forum have already been sown by the APA Council on Research, which is working to build a consensus on research training strategies in psychiatry that includes a broad range of stakeholders, such as NIMH, the Psychiatry RRC, and the ABPN. The council's current approach is to build a consensus on research training in psychiatry, mainly through outreach and communication (personal communication, J. Greden and M. Asher, APA Council on Research, August 2002). It is the committee's view that some actual training programs, as well as workforce assessment and outcome research, should be added to this forum's effort. Those activities would obviously require time and resources that could be furnished by NIMH, but resources should also be provided by foundations, industry, professional societies, and other entities with interest in such a consensus effort to develop best practices in psychiatric research training.

An example of a coordinated national research-training effort comes from pediatrics. More than a decade ago, seven national pediatric organizations, including the American Board of Pediatrics, the American Academy of Pediatrics, the Association of Medical School Pediatric Department Chairs, and the Association of Pediatric Program Directors, created the Federation of Pediatric Organizations and began meeting twice annually to deliberate issues of mutual concern and interest. Following the publication of a report on the future of pediatric education, the federation formed a standing group, the Pediatric Education Committee, to implement the recommendations of that report (Simon et al., 2000). That committee, which has research requirements as a major agenda item, is supported financially by contributions from all parent societies and has a budget to fund a national director and office.

Although such planning and evaluation require resources, it is the committee's impression that a considerable amount of data can be collected with slight modification to data collection efforts already in place at NIMH (through the grant application system) and the Accreditation Council for Graduate Medical Education (ACGME) (through the accreditation process). These datasets could be mined on a regular basis to determine programmatic and individual successes regarding research productivity and research training. The proposed coordinating body could help identify what variables will be most useful for review in an effort to determine how best to evaluate patient-oriented research training in U.S. psychiatry. Finally, it should be reiterated here that psychiatry, in working to increase its presence in patient-oriented research, should collaborate closely with other mental health practitioners and researchers who share the field's professional goals and who furthermore have historically been extremely valuable colleagues and mentors to psychiatrist-researchers.

Another resource and potential model for a national body focused on research training in psychiatry is the Institute of Medicine's (IOM) Clinical Research Roundtable. The roundtable brings together leaders across academic medicine—including university, government, and industry clinical administrators and researchers—to discuss ways of promoting clinical research. It hosts seminars on clinical research and maintains a website that links researchers at all levels to funding sources and other information about clinical research careers. The roundtable is also involved in data collection efforts (e.g., surveys and focus groups) aimed at characterizing the size and scope of the clinical research workforce (IOM, 2002a; Sung et al., 2003).

In summary, the present report characterizes the current state of research training in psychiatry and makes suggestions for enhancing this training. In carrying out its charge from NIMH, the committee was able to gather some data to support the underlying premise that more psychiatrist-researchers are necessary, but hard data in support of that contention were difficult to find. Similarly, the committee uncovered numerous descriptions, both within and outside of psychiatry, of patient-oriented or clinical research training methods. Again, however, hard data on this issue were difficult to find. Specifically, while considerable data on physician-researchers are now available, there is a paucity of data on the subgroup of patient-oriented psychiatrist-researchers. Additionally, effectiveness data are lacking on various educational approaches and how those approaches compare with one another or with nonpedagogical barriers to and incentives for research careers (e.g., personal finances, lifestyle concerns, drive). Finally, the committee was encouraged to find that many national organizations and individual departments in psychiatry are interested in enhancing early-career research training. All of these observations support the importance of establishing an ongoing national effort to develop, implement, and evaluate programs devoted to furthering that goal. Given the compelling issues posed by mental illness and the techniques now available to address those issues, such an endeavor should be exciting and rewarding for all who become involved.

References

AACAP (American Academy of Child and Adolescent Psychiatry). 2002a. *AACAP/Pfizer Travel Grants*. [Online]. Available: http://www.aacap.org/web/aacap/awards/announcm.htm [accessed January 7, 2003].

AACAP. 2002b. *AACAP Work Force Data Sheet: Critical Shortage of Child and Adolescent Psychiatrists*. [Online]. Available: http://www.aacap.org/training/workforce.htm [accessed January 7, 2003].

AACAP. 2002c. *Eli Lilly 2002 General Resident Fellows Program*. [Online]. Available: http://www.aacap.org/web/aacap/awards/lillyTravel.htm [accessed January 7, 2003].

AACAP. 2002d. *Jeanne Spurlock Research Fellowship in Drug Abuse and Addiction for Minority Medical Students*. [Online]. Available: http://www.aacap.org/web/aacap/research/spurlck1.htm [accessed January 7, 2003].

AACAP. 2003a. *Early Investigators Group*. [Online]. Available: http://www.aacap.org/research/eig.htm [accessed January 7, 2003].

AACAP. 2003b. *Integrating Training Programs in Child, Adolescent, and Adult Psychiatry*. Washington, DC: AACAP

AADPRT (American Association of Directors of Psychiatric Residency Training). 2003. *International Medical Graduate Mentorship Program in Psychiatry Program Description*. [Online]. Available: http://www.aadprt.org/public/IMG_2003/program_description.html [accessed April 9, 2003].

AAMC (Association of American Medical Colleges). 1996. *Enhancing the Environment for Women in Academic Medicine: Resources and Pathways*. Washington, DC: AAMC.

AAMC. 1999. *For the Health of the Public: Ensuring the Future of Clinical Research*. Washington, DC: AAMC

AAMC. 2001. *"All-Payer" GME Trust Fund Legislation*. [Online]. Available: http://www.aamc.org/advocacy/library/gme/gme0011.htm [accessed January 7, 2003].

AAMC. 2002a. *2002 Medical School Graduation Questionnaire All School Report*. Washington, DC: AAMC

AAMC. 2002b. *AAMC Data Book : Statistical Information Related to Medical Education*. Washington, DC: AAMC.

AAMC. 2002c. *Medical School Debt Fact Card*. [Online]. Available: www.aamc.org/students/financing/debthelp/factcard02.pdf [accessed April 8, 2003].

AAMC. 2002d. *Schools Offering Combined Degree Programs in MD/MPH*. [Online]. Available: http://services.aamc.org/currdir/section3/degree-

2.cfm?data=yes&program=mdmph [accessed March 21, 2003].
AAMC. 2003. *AAMC Responds to Residents' Lawsuit.* [Online]. Available: http://www.aamc.org/newsroom/jungcomplaint/start.htm [accessed July 10, 2003].
ABIM (American Board of Internal Medicine). 2002. *Policy and Requirements for Research Training and Certification.* [Online]. Available: http://www.abim.org/subspec/pathway/preface.htm [accessed December 18, 2002].
ABP (American Board of Pediatrics). 2001. *American Board of Pediatrics Special Alternative Pathway.* [Online]. Available: http://www.abp.org/certinfo/genpeds/sap.htm [accessed January 5, 2003].
ABP. 2002a. *The American Board of Pediatrics: Proposed Revised Requirements for Subspecialty Training.* [Online]. Available: http://www.abp.org/frtrain.htm [accessed January 2, 2003].
ABP. 2002b. *American Board of Pediatrics Subspecialty "Fast Tracking".* [Online]. Available: http://www.abp.org/frsubpol.htm [accessed January 5, 2003].
ABPN (American Board of Psychiatry and Neurology). 2002. *Part I Psychiatry Examination: Psychiatry Content Outline.* [Online]. Available: www.abpn.com/certification/psych-psych_items.html [accessed December 31, 2002].
ABPN. 2003a. *Joint Certification Programs.* [Online]. Available: http://www.abpn.com/certification/joint.html [accessed March 9, 2003].
ABPN. 2003b. *Welcome and Introduction: American Board of Psychiatry and Neurology.* [Online]. Available: http://www.abpn.com/home.html [accessed January 5, 2003].
ACGME (Accreditation Council for Graduate Medical Education). 1995a. *Program Requirements for Residency Training in Addiction Psychiatry.* [Online]. Available: http://www.acgme.org/req/401pr795.asp [accessed March 18, 2002].
ACGME. 1995b. *Program Requirements for Residency Training in Geriatric Psychiatry.* [Online]. Available: http://www.acgme.org/req/407pr-795.asp [accessed March 18, 2002].
ACGME. 1996. *Program Requirements for Residency Training in Forensic Psychiatry.* [Online]. Available: http://www.acgme.org/req/406pr-296.asp [accessed March 18, 2002].
ACGME. 1999. *Program Requirements for Residency Education in the Subspecialties of Internal Medicine .* [Online]. Available: ftp://www.acgme.org/RRC_progReq/140sub_pr799.pdf [accessed March 12, 2003].
ACGME. 2000a. *Program Requirements for Residency Education in Child and Adolescent Psychiatry.* [Online]. Available: www.acgme.org/req/405-pr101.asp [accessed April 4, 2002].
ACGME. 2000b. *Program Requirements for Residency Training in Psychiatry.* [Online]. Available: www.acgme.org/req/400pr101.asp [accessed April 4, 2002].
ACGME. 2002a. *ACGME Homepage.* [Online]. Available: www.acgme.org [ac-

cessed April 10, 2002].
ACGME. 2002b. *ACGME: Outcome Project Descriptions*. [Online]. Available: http://www.acgme.org/outcome/project/proHome.asp [accessed December 30, 2002].
ACGME. 2002c. *ACGME Manual of Policies and Procedures for Graduate Medical Education Committees*. [Online]. Available: http://www.acgme.org/GmeDir/PPmanual902.pdf [accessed October 16, 2002].
Ahrens EH. 1992. *The Crisis in Clinical Research: Overcoming Institutional Obstacles*. New York: Oxford University Press.
Albritton TA, Fincher RM. 1997. Student interest groups: A practical and affordable way to expose students to internal medicine early in their medical school training. *American Journal of Medicine* 103(5): 337–338.
American Board of Dermatology. 2003. *Booklet of Information*. [Online]. Available: http://www.abderm.org/docs/pdf/BookOfInfo.pdf [accessed April 23, 2003].
American College of Psychiatrists. 2002. *Psychiatry Resident In-Training Examination*. [Online]. Available: http://www.acpsych.org/prite/prite.html [accessed December 30, 2002].
Anderson GF, Greenberg GD, Wynn BO. 2001. Graduate medical education: The policy debate. *Annual Review of Public Health* 22(1): 35–47.
Andreasen NC. 2001. Diversity in psychiatry: Or, why did we become psychiatrists? *American Journal of Psychiatry* 158(5): 673–675.
Andrews NC. 2002. The other physician-scientist problem: Where have all the young girls gone? *Nature Medicine* 8(5): 439–441.
APA(American Psychiatric Association). 1997a. *Directory of Psychiatry Residency Training Programs*. 7th ed. Washington, DC: APA.
APA. 1997b. *The International Psychiatrist Newsletter*. [Online]. Available: http://www.psych.org/pract_of_psych/ipnews97_5.cfm [accessed April 9, 2003].
APA. 2002a. *Application Guidelines for the APIRE/Lilly Psychiatric Research Fellowship* . [Online]. Available: http://www.psych.org/res_res/lilly-.cfm [accessed January 7, 2003].
APA. 2002b. *Description of the American Psychiatric Association*. [Online]. Available: http://www.psych.org/aboutapa.cfm [accessed April 11, 2002].
APA. 2002c. Evaluation Summary: Responses from Survey of 177 Colloquium Participants.
APA. 2002d. *Program for Minority Research Training in Psychiatry (PMRTP)*. [Online]. Available: http://www.psych.org/res_res/pmrtp5302.cfm [accessed June 19, 2002].
APA. 2003. *Request for Nominations APA's Research Colloquium for Junior Investigators*. [Online]. Available: http://www.psych.org/res_res/2003-nomcolloquium62002.doc [accessed January 7, 2003].
Appelbaum AS, Stone WE, Johnson JH, Heck DH. 1978. Research training in psychiatric residency programs: A survey. *Texas Reports on Biology*

and Medicine 36: 17–23.
Arcidiacono P, Nicholson SM. Unpublished. *Peer Effects in Medical School.* Available: http://hc.wharton.upenn.edu/nicholson/pdf/peereffect.pdf [accessed April 14, 2003]
Association for Patient Oriented Research. 2000. *Association for Patient Oriented Research Definition.* [Online]. Available: http://bret.mc.vanderbilt.edu/APOR/html/about.htm [accessed April 30, 2002].
Baer LD, Konrad TR, Miller JS. 1999. The need of community health centers for international medical graduates. *American Journal of Public Health* 89(10): 1570–1574.
Baer LD, Ricketts TC, Konrad TR, Mick SS. 1998. Do international medical graduates reduce rural physician shortages? *Medical Care* 36(11): 1534–1544.
Balon R, Kuhn T. 2001. Structure vs. laissez-faire: Master of science psychiatry program and other aspects of the Detroit experience. *Academic Psychiatry* 25(1): 61–67.
Balon R, Munoz RA, Rao NR. 1999. The international medical graduate in American psychiatry. In: Weissman SH, Sabshin M, Eist H, eds. *Psychiatry in the New Millenium.* 1st ed. Washington, DC: APA. Pp. 285–299.
Balon R, Singh S. 2001. Status of research training in psychiatry. *Academic Psychiatry* 25(1): 34–41.
Barrom CP, Shadish WR, Montgomery LM. 1988. PhDs, PsyDs, and real-world constraints on scholarly activity: Another look at the boulder method. *Professional Psychology–Research and Practice* 19(1): 93–101.
Barton S, ed. 2000. *Clinical Evidence (Issue 4).* London: BMJ Publishing Group.
Batalden P, Leach D, Swing S, Dreyfus H, Dreyfus S. 2002. General competencies and accreditation in graduate medical education. *Health Affairs* 21(5): 103–111.
Beck AT. 1993. Cognitive therapy: Past, present, and future. *Journal of Consulting and Clinical Psychology* 61(2): 194–198.
Becker GS. 1993. *Human Capital.* Chicago: University of Chicago Press.
Beitman BD, Yue D. 1999. *Learning Psychotherapy: A Time-Efficient, Research-Based, and Outcome-Measured Training Program.* New York: W.W. Norton & Company.
Belar CD, Perry NW. 1992. National conference on scientist-practitioner education and training for the professional practice of psychology. *American Psychologist* 47(1): 71–75.
Beresin EV. 1997. Child and adolescent psychiatry residency training: Current issues and controversies. *Journal of the American Academy of Child and Adolescent Psychiatry* 36(10): 1339–1348.
Beresin EV, Borus JF. 1989. Child psychiatry fellowship training: A crisis in recruitment and manpower. *American Journal of Psychiatry* 146(6): 759–763.
Berg D, Cerletty J, Byrd JC. 1993. The impact of educational loan burden on

housestaff career decisions. *Journal of General Internal Medicine* 8(3): 143–145.

Bertolino A, Weinberger DR. 1999. Proton magnetic resonance spectroscopy in schizophrenia. *European Journal of Radiology* 30(2): 132–141.

Bickel J, Clark V, Lawson RM. 2002a. *Women in U.S. Academic Medicine Statistics 2001–2002*. [Online]. Available: http://www.aamc.org/members/wim/resources.htm [accessed January 9, 2003].

Bickel J, Wara D, Atkinson BF, Cohen LS, Dunn M, Hostler S, Johnson TR, Morahan P, Rubenstein AH, Sheldon GF, Stokes E. 2002b. Increasing women's leadership in academic medicine: Report of the AAMC Project Implementation Committee. *Academic Medicine* 77(10): 1043–1061.

Blake DJ, Lezotte DC, Yablon S, Rondinelli RD. 1994. Structured research training in residency training programs. The impact on the level of resident research activity. *American Journal of Physical Medicine & Rehabilitation* 73(4): 245–250.

Blazer DG, Hays JC, eds. 1998. *An Introduction to Clinical Research in Psychiatry*. New York: Oxford University Press.

Borkovec TD, Ruscio AM. 2001. Psychotherapy for generalized anxiety disorder. *Journal of Clinical Psychiatry* 62 (111): 37–42.

Brainard J. 2002. Have-nots seek more funds from the NIH. *The Chronicle of Higher Education* : A23–A24.

Braslow JT. 2002 (September 26). *Psychiatric Science and Therapeutics in the Twentieth Century*. Paper Presented at the Institute of Medicine Committee on Incorporating Research into Psychiatry Residency Training. Woods Hole, MA.

British Broadcasting Company. 2002. *TV rapped over 'cartoon therapists'*. [Online]. Available: http://news.bbc.co.uk/2/hi/health/1672292.stm [accessed July 15, 2003].

Brotherton SE, Simon FE, Etzel SI. 2002. U.S. graduate medical education, 2001–2002: Changing dynamics. *Journal of the American Medical Association* 288(9): 1073–1078.

Bruce ML. 2002 (October). *Career outcomes of entry level NIMH career awards in geriatric psychiatry*. Career Development and Training in Geriatric Mental Health. Rockville, MD.

Bureau of Labor Statistics. 2002. *2001 National Occupational Employment and Wage Estimates for Psychiatrists*. [Online]. Available: http://www.bls.gov/oes/2001/oes291066.htm [accessed March 3, 2003].

Caspi A, Sugden K, Moffitt TE, Taylor A, Craig IW, Harrington H, McClay J, Mill J, Martin J, Braithwaite A, Poulton R. 2003. Influence of life stress on depression: Moderation by a polymorphism in the 5-HTT gene. *Science* 301(5631): 386–389.

Centers for Disease Control and Prevention. 2002. *Epidemic Intelligence Service: Program Overview*. [Online]. Available: http://www.cdc.gov/eis/applyeis/applyeis.htm [accessed April 18, 2003].

Chambless DL, Ollendick TH. 2001. Empirically supported psychological inter-

ventions: Controversies and evidence. *Annual Review of Psychology* 52: 685–716.
Charney DS, Bunney BS, Nestler EJ, eds. 2001. *Neurobiology of Mental Illness*. New York: Oxford University Press.
Chen C, Balogh M, Bathija J, Howanitz E, Plutchik R, Conte HR. 1992. Substance abuse among psychiatric inpatients. *Comprehensive Psychiatry* 33(1): 60–64.
Chin D, Hopkins D, Melmon K, Holman HR. 1985. The relation of faculty academic activity to financing sources in a department of medicine. *New England Journal of Medicine* 312(16): 1029–1034.
Clayton AH, Sheldon-Keller AE. 2001. The design and evaluation of a group research experience during psychiatric residency training. *Academic Psychiatry* 25(1): 68–76.
Clayton PJ. 2002 (June 19). *Obstacles to Clinical M.D. Research from a Chairman's Point of View*. Presentation at the Institute of Medicine Workshop of the Committee on Incorporating Research into Psychiatry Residency Training. Washington, DC.
Clothier JL, Freeman T, Snow L. 2001. Medical student attitudes and knowledge about ECT. *Journal of ECT* 17(2): 99–101.
CME (Council on Medical Education). 2003. *Final Actions of the Council on Medical Education Reports and Resolutions at the Annual 2002 Meeting of the AMA House of Delegates*. [Online]. Available: http://www.ama-assn.org/ama/pub/category/2959.html [accessed January 3, 2003].
COGME (Council on Graduate Medical Education). 1998. *Summary of Eleventh Report*. [Online]. Available: http://www.cogme.gov/rpt11.htm [accessed April 9, 2003].
COGME. 2000. *Evaluation of Specialty Physician Workforce Methodologies*. Rockville, MD: Health Resources and Service Administration, DHHS
Colquitt WL, Zeh MC, Killian CD, Cultice JM. 1996. Effect of debt on U.S. medical school graduates' preferences for family medicine, general internal medicine, and general pediatrics. *Academic Medicine* 71(4): 399–411.
Columbia University. 2002. *Department of Psychiatry Columbia University*. [Online]. Available: http://cpmcnet.columbia.edu/dept/pi/psychres/welc.html [accessed November 13, 2002].
Commonwealth Fund Taskforce on Academic Health Centers. 1999. *From Bench to Bedside: Preserving the Research Mission of AHCs*. New York: Commonwealth Fund
Corsico A, McGuffin P. 2001. Psychiatric genetics: Recent advances and clinical implications. *Epidemiologia e Psichiatria Sociale* 10(4): 253–259.
Costa ST, Ausiello D, Joiner K, Neilson EG, Taylor I, Wenzel R. 2000. Supporting research in Departments of Internal Medicine: Recommendations for NIH. *American Journal of Medicine* 109(2): 178–180.
Cull WL, Mulvey HJ, O'Connor KG, Sowell DR, Berkowitz CD, Britton CV. 2002. Pediatricians working part-time: Past, present, and future. *Pedi-*

atrics 109(6): 1015–1020.

Culliton BJ. 1984. NIH starts review of training programs. *Science* 223(4632): 149–150.

Curry C. 1997. Strategies for enhancing research and research training programs for African Americans: Viewing barriers as opportunities. *Journal of Health Care for the Poor and Underserved* 8(3): 318–321.

Davis WK, Kelley WN. 1982. Factors influencing decisions to enter careers in clinical investigation. *Journal of Medical Education* 57(4): 275–281.

Dawkins K. 2002 (June 19). *Reflections/Comments from Current and Former Training Directors*. Presentation at the Institute of Medicine Workshop of the Committee on Incorporating Research into Psychiatry Residency Training. Washington, DC.

Decade of Behavior. 2001. *Behavior Matters: How Research Improves Our Lives*. [Online]. Available: www.decadeofbehavior.org [accessed January 17, 2003].

DeHaven MJ, Wilson GR, O'Connor-Kettlestrings P. 1998. Creating a research culture: What we can learn from residencies that are successful in research. *Family Medicine* 30(7): 501–507.

DHHS (U.S. Department of Health and Human Services). 1999. *Mental Health: A Report of the Surgeon General*. Washington, DC: DHHS

DHHS. 2000. *Report of the Surgeon General's Conference on Children's Mental Health: A National Action Agenda*. Washington, DC: DHHS

DHHS. 2001a. *Mental Health: Culture, Race, and Ethnicity–A Supplement to Mental Health: A Report of the Surgeon General*. Rockville, MD: DHHS, Substance Abuse and Mental Health Services Administration, Center for Mental Health Services, National Institutes of Health, National Institute of Mental Health

DHHS. 2001b. *Women and Smoking: A Report of the Surgeon General*. Rockville, MD: DHHS

DHHS. 2001c. *Youth Violence: A Report of the Surgeon General*. Rockville, MD: DHHS

DHHS. 2002. *Reducing Tobacco Use: A Report of the Surgeon General*. Rockville, MD: DHHS

Dial T, Haviland MG, Pincus HA. 1990. Factors associated with future psychiatrists' selection of academic or clinical careers. *Academic Psychiatry* 14: 164–171.

Doherty MJ, Schneider AT, Tirschwell DL. 2002. Will neurology residents with large student loan debts become academicians? *Neurology* 58(3): 495–497.

Drell MJ. 2002 (June 19). *Reflections/Comments from Current and Former Training Directors*. Presentation at the Institute of Medicine Workshop of the Committee on Incorporating Research into Psychiatry Residency Training. Washington, DC.

Dunn JC, Lai EC, Brooks CM, Stabile BE, Fonkalsrud EW. 1998. The outcome of research training during surgical residency. *Journal of Pediatric Surgery* 33(2): 362–364.

Durston S, Hulshoff Pol HE, Casey BJ, Giedd JN, Buitelaar JK, van Engeland H. 2001. Anatomical MRI of the developing human brain: What have we learned? *Journal of the American Academy of Child and Adolescent Psychiatry* 40(9): 1012–1020.

Eisenberg L. 2002. Themes in twentieth century American psychiatry. In: Hager M, ed. *Modern Psychiatry: Challenges in Educating Health Professionals to Meet New Needs. A Conference Sponsored by the Josiah Macy, Jr. Foundation*. New York: Josiah Macy, Jr. Foundation. Pp. 30–62.

Emory School of Medicine. 2000. *Clinical Research Curriculum Award Program at Emory University*. [Online]. Available: http://www.sph.emory-.edu/CRCA/ [accessed March 20, 2003].

Fang D, Meyer RE. 2003. PhD faculty in clinical departments of U.S. medical schools, 1981-1999: Their widening presence and roles in research. *Academic Medicine* 78(2): 167–176.

Feifel D, Moutier CY, Swerdlow NR. 1999. Attitudes toward psychiatry as a prospective career among students entering medical school. *American Journal of Psychiatry* 156(9): 1397–1402.

Fenton WS. 2002 (April 12). *Sponsor Presentation of Study Genesis and Charge*. Presentation at the Institute of Medicine Committee on Incorporating Research into Psychiatry Residency Training. Washington, DC.

Fishman DB, Zimet CN. 1972. Specialty choice and beliefs about specialties among freshman medical students. *Journal of Medical Education* 47(7): 524–533.

Fitz-Gerald MJ, Kablinger A, Manno B, Carter OS, Caldito G, Smith S. 2001. Psychiatry residents' participation in research: A survey of attitudes and experience. *Academic Psychiatry* 25(1): 42–47.

Foa EB, Keane T, Friedman MJ, eds. 2000. *Effective Treatments for PTSD: Practice Guidelines from the International Society for Traumatic Stress Studies*. New York: Guilford Press.

Frank E, Boswell L, Dickstein L, Chapman D. 2001a. Characteristics of female psychiatrists. *American Journal of Psychiatry* 158(2): 205–212.

Frank RG, Goldman HH, McGuire TG. 2001b. Will parity in coverage result in better mental health care? *New England Journal of Medicine* 345(23): 1701–1704.

Frieden C, Fox BJ. 1991. Career choices of graduates from Washington University's Medical Scientist Training Program. *Academic Medicine* 66(3): 162–164.

Friedman RM, Katz-Levey JW, Manderscheid RW, Sondheimer DL. 1996. Prevalence of serious emotional disturbance in children and adolescents. In: Manderscheid RW, Sonnenschein MA, eds. *Mental Health, United States, 1996*. Rockville, MD: Center for Mental Health Services. Pp. 71–78.

Fu CH, McGuire PK. 1999. Functional neuroimaging in psychiatry. *Philosophical Transactions of the Royal Society of London – Series B: Biological*

Sciences 354(1387): 1359–1370.
Gabbard GO, Gunderson JG, Fonagy P. 2002. The place of psychoanalytic treatments within psychiatry. *Archives of General Psychiatry* 59(6): 505–510.
Goldman C, Williams V. 2001. *Benefits and Feasibility of a Conceptual Framework for Biomedical and Behavioral Science Personnel.* Arlington, VA: RAND
Goldman H. 2002. Improving access to evidence-based services: Translating need into supply and demand. In: Hager M, ed. *Modern Psychiatry: Challenges in Educating Health Professionals to Meet New Needs. A Conference Sponsored by the Josiah Macy, Jr. Foundation.* New York: Josiah Macy, Jr. Foundation. Pp. 93–114.
Griggs RC. 2002 (June 19). *Recruitment, Development, and Retention of Clinical Neuroscientists in Residency Training: Neurology's Perspective.* Presentation at the Institute of Medicine Workshop of the Committee on Incorporating Research into Psychiatry Residency Training. Washington, DC.
Guerra EA, Regier DA, eds. 2001. *Directory of Research Fellowship Opportunities in Psychiatry.* Washington, DC: APA
Halpain M, Jeste D, Katz I, Reynolds C, Small G, Borson S, Lebowitz B. 2001. Summer research institute: Enhancing research career development in geriatric psychiatry. *Academic Psychiatry* 25(1): 48–56.
Hamburg B. 2002. Chairman's summary of the conference. In: Hager M, ed. *Modern Psychiatry: Challenges in Educating Health Professionals to Meet New Needs. A Conference Sponsored by the Josiah Macy, Jr. Foundation.* New York: Josiah Macy, Jr. Foundation. Pp. 16–25.
Haviland MG, Pincus HA, Dial TH. 1987. Career, research involvement, and research fellowship plans of potential psychiatrists. *Archives of General Psychiatry* 44(5): 493–496.
HayGroup. 1999. *Health Care Plan Design and Cost Trends–1988 through 1998.* Arlington, VA: HayGroup
Hebert RS, Levine RB, Smith CG, Wright SM. 2003. A systematic review of resident research curricula. *Academic Medicine* 78(1): 61–68.
Henderson L, Lee B, Marino A. 2001. *Final Report on Three Focus Groups with Early Career Clinical Researchers about the K23 Award Program.* Washington, DC: AAMC
Henderson T. 2000. *Graduate Medical Education and Public Policy: A Primer.* Washington, DC: DHHS
Hendren RL, De Backer I, Pandina GJ. 2000. Review of neuroimaging studies of child and adolescent psychiatric disorders from the past 10 years. *Journal of the American Academy of Child and Adolescent Psychiatry* 39(7): 815–828.
Holmes EW, Burks TF, Dzau V, Hindery MA, Jones RF, Kaye CI, Korn D, Limbird LE, Marchase RB, Perlmutter R, Sanfilippo F, Strom BL. 2000. Measuring contributions to the research mission of medical schools. *Academic Medicine* 75(3): 303–313.

Hostetter MK. 2002. Career development for physician-scientists: The model of the Pediatric Scientist Development Program. *Journal of Pediatrics* 140(2): 143–144.

Hoyert DL, Kochanek KD, Murphy SL. 1999. Deaths: Final data for 1997. *National Vital Statistics Reports* 47(19): 1–104.

Hyman SE. 2001 (November 7). *Keynote Presentation*. National Institute of Mental Health and the American Psychiatric Association Workshop on Research Training for Psychiatrists. Bethesda, MD.

Hyman SE. 2002a. Integrating neuroscience, behavioral science and genetics in model psychiatry. In: Hager M, ed. *Modern Psychiatry: Challenges in Educating Health Professionals to Meet New Needs. A Conference Sponsored by the Josiah Macy, Jr. Foundation*. New York: Josiah Macy, Jr. Foundation. Pp. 115–131.

Hyman SE. 2002b (June 18). *Obstacles to Residency-based Research Training in Psychiatry*. Presentation at the Institute of Medicine Committee on Incorporating Research into Psychiatry Residency Training. Washington, DC.

Hyman SE, Fenton WS. 2003. Medicine. What are the right targets for psychopharmacology? *Science* 299(5605): 350–351.

IOM (Institute of Medicine). 1994. *Career in Clinical Research Obstacles and Opportunities*. Washington, DC: National Academy Press.

IOM. 2000. *Bridging Disciplines in the Brain, Behavioral, and Clinical Sciences*. Washington, DC: National Academy Press.

IOM. 2001a. *Crossing the Quality Chasm: A New Health System for the 21st Century*. Washington, DC: National Academy Press.

IOM. 2001b. *The Right Thing to Do, the Smart Thing to Do: Enhancing Diversity in Health Professions – Summary of the Symposium on Diversity in Health Professions in Honor of Herbert W. Nickens, M.D*. Washington, D.C: National Academy Press.

IOM. 2002a. *Clinical Research Roundtable*. [Online]. Available: http://www.iom.edu/IOM/IOMHome.nsf/Pages/Clinical+Research+Roundtable [accessed October 17, 2002].

IOM. 2002b. *The Role of Purchasers and Payers in the Clinical Research Enterprise: Workshop Summary*. Washington, DC: National Academy Press.

IOM. 2003. *Unequal Treatment: Confronting Racial and Ethnic Disparities in Health Care*. Washington, DC: National Academy Press.

ISI Thomson. 2001a. *Interview with Dr. Kenneth Davis of the Mount Sinai School of Medicine in New York City*. [Online]. Available: http://esi-topics.com/schizophrenia/interviews/dr-kenneth-davis.html [accessed July 11, 2002].

ISI Thomson. 2001b. *Interview with Dr. Peter McGuffin, Director of the Social, Genetic, and Developmental Psychiatric Research Centre at King's College, London*. [Online]. Available: http://www.esi-topics.com/schizophrenia/interviews/dr-peter-mcguffin.html [accessed July 11, 2002].

ISI Thomson. 2003. *ScienceWatch*. [Online]. Available: http://www.sciencewatch.com [accessed June 25, 2003].
Jacobs SC, Hoge MA, Sledge WH, Bunney BS. 1997. Managed care, health care reform, and academic psychiatry. *Academic Psychiatry* 21(2): 72–85.
Johnson JC, Jayadevappa R, Taylor L, Askew A, Williams B, Johnson B. 1998. Extending the pipeline for minority physicians: A comprehensive program for minority faculty development. *Academic Medicine* 73(3): 237–244.
Jones RF, Sanderson SC. 1996. Clinical revenues used to support the academic mission of medical schools, 1992–93. *Academic Medicine* 71(3): 299–307.
Journal of the American Medical Association. 2000. Appendix II - Graduate medical education. *Journal of the American Medical Association* 284(9): 1159–1172.
Kandel ER. 1998. A new intellectual framework for psychiatry. *American Journal of Psychiatry* 155(4): 457–469.
Kandel ER. 1999. Biology and the future of psychoanalysis: A new intellectual framework for psychiatry revisited. *American Journal of Psychiatry* 156(4): 505–524.
Kandel ER, Schwartz JH, Jessell TM, ed. 2000. *Principles of Neural Science*. 4th ed. New York: McGraw-Hill.
Kane J, Honigfeld G, Singer J, Meltzer H. 1988. Clozapine for the treatment-resistant schizophrenic. A double-blind comparison with chlorpromazine. *Archives of General Psychiatry* 45(9): 789–796.
Kanigel R. 1993. *Apprentice to Genius: A Making of a Scientific Dynasty*. Baltimore, MD: Johns Hopkins University Press.
Kaplan A. 2000. Ensuring the continuation and growth of clinical researcher. *Psychiatric Times* 17(6): 1-6.
Kassebaum DG, Szenas PL. 1995. Medical students' career indecision and specialty rejection: Roads not taken. *Academic Medicine* 70(10): 937–943.
Kassebaum DG, Szenas PL, Ruffin AL, Masters DR. 1995. The research career interests of graduating medical students. *Academic Medicine* 70(9): 848–852.
Kastor JA, Mehrling MM, Mackowiak PA, Breault PW. 1997. The salary responsibility program for full-time faculty members in an academic clinical department. *Academic Medicine* 72(1): 23–29.
Katerndahl DA. 1996. Associations between departmental features and departmental scholarly activity. *Family Medicine* 28(2): 119–127.
Kim WJ, Enzer N, Bechtold D, Brooks BA, Joshi P, King C, Robinowitz C, Stubbe D, Szigethy E, Tanquay P. 2001. *Report of the AACAP Task Force on Work Force Needs. Meeting the Mental Health Needs of Children and Adolescents: Addressing the Problems of Access to Care*. Washington, DC: AACAP
Kimball HR. 1994. The training of clinical investigators: Is the ABIM Clinical Investigator Pathway adequate? *ABIM Summer Conference Report*: 69–74.

Kimball HR, Bennett JC. 1994. Training the future internal medicine subspecialist. *American Journal of Medicine* 96(6): 559–561.

Kirchner JE, Owen RR, Nordquist CR, Clardy JA. 1998. Developing clinician scientists through integrated research training in psychiatry. *Teaching and Learning in Medicine* (10): 183–187.

Klerman GL. 1989. Evaluating the efficacy of psychotherapy for depression: The USA experience. *European Archives of Psychiatry and Neurological Sciences* 238(5-6): 240–246.

Knapp R. 2002. Complexity and uncertainty in financing graduate medical education. *Academic Medicine* 77(11): 1076–1083.

Kruse JE, Bradley J, Wesley RM, Markwell SJ. 2003. Research support infrastructure and productivity in U. S. family practice residency programs. *Academic Medicine* 78(1): 54–60.

Kupfer DJ, Hyman SE, Schatzberg AF, Pincus HA, Reynolds CF. 2002. Recruiting and retaining future generations of physician scientists in mental health. *Archives of General Psychiatry* 59(7): 657–660.

Lambert M. 2001. The status of empirically supported therapies: Comment on Weston and Morrison's (2001) Multidimensional Meta-Analysis. *Journal of Consulting and Clinical Psychology* 69(6): 910–913.

Lambert MT, Garver DL. 1998. Mentoring psychiatric trainees' first paper for publication. *Academic Psychiatry* 22(1): 47–55.

Lawson WB. 1996. The art and science of the psychopharmacotherapy of African Americans. *Mount Sinai Journal of Medicine* 63(5-6): 301–305.

Lawson WB. 2000. Issues in the pharmacotherapy of African Americans. *Review of Psychiatry* 19(4): 37–53.

Ledley FD, Lovejoy FH. 1993. Factors influencing the interest, career paths, and research activities of recent graduates from an academic, pediatric residency program. *Pediatrics* 92(3): 436–441.

Lee EK, Kaltreider N, Crouch J. 1995. Pilot study of current factors influencing the choice of psychiatry as a specialty. *American Journal of Psychiatry* 152(7): 1066–1069.

Lee TH, Ognibene FP, Schwartz JS. 1991. Correlates of external research support among respondents to the 1990 American Federation for Clinical Research Survey. *Clinical Research* 39(2): 135–44.

Leebens PK, Walker DE, Leckman JF. 1993. Determinants of academic survival: Survey of AACAP poster authors. *Journal of the American Academy of Child and Adolescent Psychiatry* 32(2): 453–461.

Leibenluft E, Dial TH, Haviland MG, Pincus HA. 1993. Sex differences in rank attainment and research activities among academic psychiatrists. *Archives of General Psychiatry* 50(11): 896–904.

Leichsenring F, Leibing E. 2003. The effectiveness of psychodynamic therapy and cognitive behavior therapy in the treatment of personality disorders: A meta-analysis. *American Journal of Psychiatry* 160(7): 1223–1232.

Leon CA. 1979. Therapeutic effects of clozapine. A 4-year follow-up of a controlled clinical trial. *Acta Psychiatrica Scandinavica* 59(5): 471–480.

Levey GS. 1992. Internal medicine and the training of international medical graduates: A time for open discussion and new approaches. *Annals of Internal Medicine* 117(5): 403–407.

Levey GS, Sherman CR, Gentile NO, Hough LJ, Dial TH, Jolly P. 1988. Postdoctoral research training of full-time faculty in academic departments of medicine. *Annals of Internal Medicine* 109(5): 414–418.

Lewinsohn PM, Gotlib IH, Hautzinger M. 1998. Behavioral treatment of unipolar depression. In: Caballo VE, ed. *International Handbook of Cognitive and Behavioural Treatments for Psychological Disorders*. 1st ed. New York: Pergamon. Pp. 441–488.

Ley TJ, Rosenberg LE. 2002. Removing career obstacles for young physician-scientists – loan-repayment programs. *New England Journal of Medicine* 346(5): 368–372.

Library of Congress. 2000. *Project on the Decade of the Brain*. [Online]. Available: http://lcweb.loc.gov/loc/brain/ [accessed September 9, 2002].

Lieberman J. 2001. Starting a career in psychiatric research. *Academic Psychiatry* 25(1): 28–30.

Ludmerer KM. 1999. *Time to Heal*. New York: Oxford University Press.

Malhi GS, Valenzuela M, Wen W, Sachdev P. 2002. Magnetic resonance spectroscopy and its applications in psychiatry. *Australian and New Zealand Journal of Psychiatry* 36(1): 31–43.

March JS. 2002 (June 19). *Research Training in Child Psychiatry*. Presentation at the Institute of Medicine Workshop for the Committee on Incorporating Research into Psychiatry Residency Training. Washington, DC.

Marder SR, May PR. 1986. Benefits and limitations of neuroleptics–and other forms of treatment–in schizophrenia. *American Journal of Psychotherapy* 40(3): 357–369.

Mavis B, Katz M. 2003. Evaluation of a program supporting scholarly productivity for new investigators. *Academic Medicine* 78(7): 757–576.

Mayo Graduate School of Medicine. 2002. *Clinician-Investigator Training Program*. [Online]. Available: http://www.mayo.edu/mgsm/ci.htm [accessed March 20, 2003].

McCullum-Smith RE. 2002. Training the next generation of biological psychiatrists: The Michigan model. *Psychiatric Research Report* 18(2): 6–7.

McGuire MT, Fairbanks LA. 1982. Research Training. In: Yager J, ed. *Teaching Psychiatry and Behavioral Science*. New York: Grune & Stratton. Pp. 243–251.

McMurray JE, Cohen M, Angus G, Harding J, Gavel P, Horvath J, Paice E, Schmittdiel J, Grumbach K. 2002. Women in medicine: A four-nation comparison. *Journal of the American Medical Women's Association* 57(4): 185–190.

Meador-Woodruff JH. 2001 (November 7). *Residency Research Track Program (R25 Model)*. National Institute of Mental Health and the American Psychiatric Association Workshop on Research Training for Psychiatrists. Bethesda, MD.

Meador-Woodruff JH. 2002 (June 19). *Mentoring Residents Interested in Re-*

search. Presentation at the Institute of Medicine Workshop of the Committee on Incorporating Research into Psychiatry Residency Training. Washington, DC.

Mechanic D. 1998. Emerging trends in mental health policy and practice. *Health Affairs* 17(6): 82–98.

Meyer RE. 2002 (June 19). *Ensuring the Future of Clinical Research across Medical Specialties*. Presentation at the Institute of Medicine Workshop of the Committee on Incorporating Research into Psychiatry Residency Training. Washington, DC.

Meyer RE, Griner PF, Weissman J. 1998. Clinical research in medical schools: Seizing the opportunity. *Proceedings of the Association of American Physicians* 110(6): 513–520.

Meyer RE, McLaughlin CJ. 1998. The place of research in the mission of academic psychiatry. In: Meyer RE, McLaughlin CJ. *Between Mind, Brain, and Managed Care*. Washington, DC: APA. Pp. 77-96.

Millenson ML. 1998. What doctors don't know. *Washington Monthly* 30(12): 8–13.

Miller ED. 2001. Clinical investigators–the endangered species revisited. *Journal of the American Medical Association* 286(7): 845–846.

Miller FH, Greaney TL. 2003. The national resident matching program and antitrust law. *Journal of the American Medical Association* 289(7): 913–918.

Miller SI. 2002 (April 12). *The Psychiatry Residency Paths*. Presentation at the Institute of Medicine Committee on Incorporating Research into Psychiatry Residency Training. Washington, DC.

Mincer J. 1974. *Schooling, Experience, and Earnings*. New York: National Bureau of Economic Research.

Mirin SM. 2002 (June 19). *Leadership Perspectives: From the Executive's Perch*. Presentation at the Institute of Medicine Workshop of the Committee on Incorporating Research into Psychiatry Residency Training. Washington, DC.

Moresco RM, Messa C, Lucignani G, Rizzo GG, Todde S, Gilardi CM, Grimaldi A, Fazio F. 2001. PET in psychopharmacology. *Pharmacological Research* 44(3): 151–159.

Moseley JB, O'Malley K, Petersen NJ, Menke TJ, Brody BA, Kuykendall DH, Hollingsworth JC, Ashton CM, Wray NP. 2002. A controlled trial of arthroscopic surgery for osteoarthritis of the knee. *New England Journal of Medicine* 347(2): 81–88.

Moy E, Mazzaschi AJ, Levin RJ, Blake DA, Griner PF. 1997. Relationship between National Institutes of Health research awards to U.S. medical schools and managed care market penetration. *Journal of the American Medical Association* 278(3): 217–221.

Mullan F. 2000. The case for more U.S. medical students. *New England Journal of Medicine* 343(3): 213–217.

Mulrow CD, Lohr KN. 2001. Proof and policy from medical research evidence. *Journal of Health Politics, Policy and Law* 26(2): 249–266.

Murray CL, Lopez AD, eds. 1996. *The Global Burden of Disease: A Comprehensive Assessment of Mortality and Disability from Disease, Injuries, and Risk Factors in 1990 and Projected to 2020.* Cambridge, MA: Harvard University Press.

NARSAD (National Alliance for Research on Schizophrenia and Depression). 2002. *NARSAD's Young Investigator Award.* [Online]. Available: http://www.narsad.org/research/yiprogram.html [accessed March 6, 2002].

NARSAD. 2003. *2004 Guidelines NARSAD's Young Investigator Award.* [Online]. Available: http://www.narsad.org/research/yigdlns.html [accessed March 6, 2003].

Nasrallah HA. 2002 (June 19). *Overcoming Obstacles to Research in Psychiatry Residency Training.* Presentation at the Institute of Medicine Workshop of the Committee on Incorporating Research into Psychiatry Residency Training. Washington, DC.

Nathan DG. 1998. Clinical research: perceptions, reality, and proposed solutions. National Institutes of Health Director's Panel on Clinical Research. *Journal of the American Medical Association* 280(16): 1427–1431.

Nathan DG. 2002. Educational-debt relief for clinical investigators – A vote of confidence. *The New England Journal of Medicine* 346(5): 372–374.

Nathan PE, Gorman JM, eds. 1998. *A Guide to Treatments that Work.* New York: Oxford University Press.

National Advisory Mental Health Council's Workgroup on Racial/Ethnic Diversity in Research Training and Health Disparities Research. 2001. *An Investment in America's Future Racial/Ethnic Diversity in Mental Health Research Careers.* Washington, DC: DHHS

National Public Radio. 2002. *All Things Considered: Evidence Suggests Autism Begins in Genes.* [Online]. Available: http://www.npr.org/rundowns/rundown.php?prgId=2&prgDate=25-Nov-2002 [accessed May 7, 2003].

National Public Radio. 2003. *Morning Edition: DNA and the Brain.* [Online]. Available: http://www.npr.org/rundowns/rundown.php?prgId=3&prgDate=25-Apr-2003 [accessed May 7, 2003].

Neinstein LS, MacKenzie RG. 1989. Prior training and recommendations for future training of clinical research faculty members. *Academic Medicine* 64(1): 32–5.

Nemetz P, Weiner H. 1965. Some factors in the choice of psychiatry as a career. *Archives of General Psychiatry* 13(4): 299–303.

Nevin J, Pincus HA, eds. 1992. *Directory of Research Fellowship Opportunities in Psychiatry.* Washington, DC: APA

New Freedom Commission on Mental Health. 2003. *Achieving the Promise: Transforming Mental Health Care in America. Final Report.* Rockville, MD: DHHS

Newhouse J, Wilensky G. 2001. Paying for graduate medical education: The debate goes on. *Health Affairs* 20(2): 136–147.

NIAAA (National Institute of Alcohol Abuse and Alcoholism). 2002. *Notice of Funding Opportunity for Mentored Patient-Oriented Research Career Development Award (K-23)*. [Online]. Available: http://www.niaaa.nih.gov/extramural/noticek23.htm [accessed April 30, 2002].

NICHD (National Institute of Child Health and Human Development). 2002. *Scientific Director's Preface*. [Online]. Available: http://dir2.nichd.nih.gov/info/ar/a1.php3 [accessed April 30, 2002].

Nicholson SM. 2002 (June 19). *Personal Economics and Other Factors Influencing Specialty Selection*. Presentation at the Institute of Medicine Workshop of the Committee on Incorporating Research into Psychiatry Residency Training. Washington, DC.

NIH (National Institutes of Health). 1997a. *Director's Panel on Clinical Research: Executive Summary*. [Online]. Available: http://www.nih.gov/news/crp/97report/execsum.htm#2define [accessed April 30, 2002].

NIH. 1997b. *The NIH Director's Panel on Clinical Research Report to the Advisory Committee of the Director*. [Online]. Available: http://www.nih.gov/news/crp/97report/ [accessed February 12, 2002].

NIH. 1999a. *Computer Retrieval of Information on Scientific Projects (CRISP)*. [Online]. Available: http://crisp.cit.nih.gov [accessed April 9, 2002].

NIH. 1999b. *Mentored Patient-Oriented Research Career Development Award (K23)*. [Online]. Available: http://grants1.nih.gov/grants/guide/pa-files/PA-00-004.html [accessed April 22, 2003].

NIH. 1999c. *Midcareer Investigator Award in Patient-Oriented Research (K24)*. [Online]. Available: http://grants.nih.gov/grants/guide/pa-files/PA-00-005.html [accessed April 22, 2003].

NIH. 2000a. *National Research Service Award for Individual Predoctoral Fellows*. [Online]. Available: http://grants1.nih.gov/grants/guide/pa-files/PA-00-125.html [accessed December 9, 2002].

NIH. 2000b. *Request for Applications: Biomedical Research Infrastructure Network*. [Online]. Available: http://grants1.nih.gov/grants/guide/rfa-files/RFA-RR-01-005.html [accessed April 10, 2003].

NIH. 2000c. *NIMH Minority Research Infrastructure Support Program (R24)*. [Online]. Available: http://grants.nih.gov/grants/guide/pa-files/PAR-01-029.html [accessed April 22, 2003].

NIH. 2001a. *NIH Grants Policy Statement (Rev. 3/01)*. Rockville, MD: DHHS, Public Health Service, National Institutes of Health

NIH. 2001b. *Request for Applications: Centers of Biomedical Research Excellence*. [Online]. Available: http://grants1.nih.gov/grants/guide/rfa-files/RFA-RR-02-003.html [accessed April 10, 2003].

NIH. 2002a. *Office of Loan Repayment and Scholarship–NIH Loan Repayment Programs*. [Online]. Available: http://www.lrp.nih.gov/about/extramural/intro.htm [accessed April 8, 2003].

NIH. 2002b. *NIH National Research Service Award Institutional Research Training Grants (T32)*. [Online]. Available: http://grants1.nih.gov/grants/guide/pa-files/PA-02-109.html [accessed November 21, 2002].

NIH. 2002c. *Request for Applications: Centers of Biomedical Research Excel-

lence. [Online]. Available: http://grants1.nih.gov/grants/guide/rfa-files/RFA-RR-02-007.html [accessed April 10, 2003].
NIH. 2003a. *National Center for Research Resources Homepage.* [Online]. Available: http://www.ncrr.nih.gov/ [accessed April 26, 2003].
NIH. 2003b. *NIH Awards to Medical Schools by Department and Rank, FY2002.* [Online]. Available: http://grants1.nih.gov/grants/award/trends/medpt02.xls [accessed May 4, 2003].
NIH. 2003c. *Ruth L. Kirschstein National Research Service Awards for Individual Postdoctoral Fellows (F32).* [Online]. Available: http://grants1.nih.gov/grants/guide/pa-files/PA-03-067.html [accessed March 11, 2003].
NIH. 2003d. *Revision of March 7, 2003 Notice About Ruth L. Kirschstein National Research Service Award (NRSA) Stipend Increase and Other Budgetary Changes Effective for Fiscal Year 2003.* [Online]. Available: http://grants.nih.gov/grants/guide/notice-files/NOT-OD-03-036.html [accessed September 15, 2003].
NIH. 2003e. *K Kiosk: Information about NIH Career Development Awards.* [Online]. Available: http://grants1.nih.gov/training/careerdevelopmentawards.htm [accessed May 1, 2003].
NIH. 2003f. *Education Activities at the Office of Human Research Protections.* [Online]. Available: http://ohrp.osophs.dhhs.gov/educmat.htm [accessed May 1, 2003].
NIMH (National Institute of Mental Health). 1994. *Research Infrastructure Support Program (PAR-94-096).* [Online]. Available: http://www.nimh.nih.gov/grants/research/94096.cfm [accessed August 7, 2003].
NIMH. 1999. *Summary of Workshop on Underrepresented Racial/Ethnic Minority Training.* [Online]. Available: http://www.nimh.nih.gov/research/minoritytraining.pdf [accessed January 7, 2003].
NIMH. 2000a. *NIMH Training Programs for Underrepresented Racial/Ethnic Minorities: NIMH Interim Staff Report.* Rockville, MD: NIMH
NIMH. 2000b. *A Participant's Guide to Mental Health Clinical Research.* [Online]. Available: http://www.nimh.nih.gov/studies/clinres.cfm [accessed December 31, 2002].
NIMH. 2000c. *Interventions and Practice Research Infrastructure (PAR-00-096).* [Online]. Available: http://grants.nih.gov/grants/guide/pa-files/PAR-00-096.html [accessed August 7, 2003].
NIMH. 2001a. *Research Grant Application and Award Statistics.* [Online]. Available: www.nimh.nih.gov/srcbook/2000/page.cfm [accessed September 12, 2002].
NIMH. 2001b. *Science on Our Minds.* [Online]. Available: http://www.nimh.nih.gov/publicat/soms.cfm [accessed November 14, 2002].
NIMH. 2001c. *The Numbers Count: Mental Disorders in America.* [Online]. Available: http://www.nimh.nih.gov/publicat/numbers.cfm [accessed February 5, 2003].
NIMH. 2002a. *Investigator-Development Workshop for "K" Awardees and Prospective Awardees.* [Online]. Available: http://www.nimh.nih-.gov/childhp/kmeeting.htm [accessed June 13, 2002].

NIMH. 2002b. *PGY4 Psychiatric Residency Program*. [Online]. Available: http://intramural.nimh.nih.gov/training/pgy4-programexp.pdf [accessed December 10, 2002].

NIMH. 2002c. *PGY4 Residency Training Program*. [Online]. Available: http://intramural.nimh.nih.gov/training/pgy4.htm [accessed December 10, 2002].

NIMH. 2002d. *Extramural Loan Repayment Program*. [Online]. Available: http://www.nimh.nih.gov/grants/loanrepayment.cfm [accessed April 8, 2003].

Nolan J, Beaulieu M, Puccio K, Forte G, Salsberg E. 2002. *Residency Training Outcomes by Specialty in 2001 for New York State: A Summary of Responses to the 2001 NYS Resident Exit Survey*. Rensselaer, NY: University at Albany, State University of New York

Nolan J, Forte G, Salsberg E. 2003. *Physician Supply and Demand Indicators in New York and California: A Summary of Trends in Starting Income, Relative Demand, and GME Graduates in 35 Medical Specialties*. Rensselaer, NY: University at Albany, State University of New York

NRC (National Research Council). 1997. *Advisor, Teacher, Role Model, Friend: On Being a Mentor to Students in Science and Engineering*. Washington, DC: National Academy Press.

NRC. 2000. *Addressing the Nation's Changing Needs for Biomedical and Behavioral Scientists*. Washington, DC: National Academy Press.

Oinonen MJ, Crowley WF, Moskowitz J, Vlasses PH. 2001. How do academic health centers value and encourage clinical research? *Academic Medicine* 76(7): 700–706.

Olfson M, Marcus SC, Pincus HA. 1999. Trends in office-based psychiatric practice. *American Journal of Psychiatry* 156(3): 451–457.

Osborn EH, Ernster VL, Martin JB. 1992. Women's attitudes toward careers in academic medicine at the University of California, San Francisco. *Academic Medicine* 67(1): 59–62.

Paiva RE, Haley HB. 1971. Intellectual, personality, and environmental factors in career specialty preferences. *Journal of Medical Education* 46(4): 281–289.

Paniagua FA, Pumariega AJ, O'Boyle M, Meyer WJ. 1993. The role of a research seminar for child psychiatry residents. *Journal of the American Academy of Child and Adolescent Psychiatry* 32(2): 446–452.

Pardes H. 2002 (June 18). *Obstacles to Integrating Research into Residency Training*. Presentation at the Institute of Medicine Committee on Incorporating Research into Psychiatry Residency Training. Washington, DC.

Pardes H, Pincus HA. 1983. Challenges to academic psychiatry. *American Journal of Psychiatry* 140(9): 1117–1126.

Pasko T, Seidman B. 2002. *Physician Characteristics and Distribution in the U.S. 2002–2003 Edition*. Chicago: AMA.

Pato M, Pato C. 2001. Teaching research basics to all residents: Ten years of experience. *Academic Psychiatry* 25(1): 77–81.

Pincus HA, ed. 1995. *Research Funding and Resource Manual Mental Health and Addictive Disorders*. 1st ed. Washington, DC: APA.
Pincus HA. 2001a (November 7). *Residency Research Track Program (R25 Model)*. National Institute of Mental Health and the American Psychiatric Association Workshop on Research Training for Psychiatrists. Bethesda, MD.
Pincus HA. 2001b. Preserving the psychiatrist-investigator. *Academic Psychiatry* 25(1): 15-16.
Pincus HA. 2002 (June 18). *Obstacles to Integrating Research into Residency Training*. Presentation at the Institute of Medicine Committee on Incorporating Research into Psychiatry Residency Training. Washington, DC.
Pincus HA, Dial TH, Haviland MG. 1993. Research activities of full-time faculty in academic departments of psychiatry. *Archives of General Psychiatry* 50(8): 657-664.
Pincus HA, Haviland MG, Dial TH, Hendryx MS. 1995. The relationship of postdoctoral research training to current research activities of faculty in academic departments of psychiatry. *American Journal of Psychiatry* 152(4): 596-601.
Pinker S. 2003. Are your genes to blame? *Time* 161(3): 98-100.
Pottick KJ, McAlpine DD, Andelman RB. 2000. Changing patterns of psychiatric inpatient care for children and adolescents in general hospitals, 1988-1995. *American Journal of Psychiatry* 157(8): 1267-1273.
Potts JT. 1992. Recruitment of minority physicians into careers in internal medicine. *Annals of Internal Medicine* 116(12 Pt 2): 1099-1102.
President's New Freedom Commission on Mental Health. 2002. *Interim Report*. [Online]. Available: http://www.mentalhealthcommission.gov/reports/Final_Interim_Report.doc [accessed November 21, 2002]
Proctor J. 2000. Medical school debt: Making sense of life in the red. *AAMC Reporter* 9(6).
Rancurello MD. 1988. Research training in psychiatry: Considerations at the preresidency level. *Psychopharmacology Bulletin* 24(2): 293-299.
Raphael B, Dunne M, Byrne G. 1990. A research seminar programme for doctoral candidates in psychiatry. *Australian and New Zealand Journal of Psychiatry* 24(2): 207-213.
Regier DA, Farmer ME, Rae DS, Locke BZ, Keith SJ, Judd LL, Goodwin FK. 1990. Comorbidity of mental disorders with alcohol and other drug abuse. Results from the Epidemiologic Catchment Area (ECA) study. *Journal of the American Medical Association* 264(19): 2511-2518.
Research!America. 2002. *Research!America 2001 Aggregate Public Opinion Poll Data*. [Online]. Available: http://researchamerica.org/opinions/2001polls.generalversion.pdf [accessed April 16, 2003].
Reynolds C, Martin C, Brent D, Ryan N, Dahl R, Pilkonis P, Marcus M, Kupfer D. 1998. Postdoctoral clinical-research training in psychiatry. *Academic Psychiatry* 22(3): 190-196.
Rieder RO. 1988. The recruitment and training of psychiatric residents for re-

search. *Psychopharmacology Bulletin* 24(2): 288–290.
Rieder RO. 2001 (November 7). *Columbia Model (T32 Model).* National Institute of Mental Health and the American Psychiatric Association Workshop on Research Training for Psychiatrists. Bethesda, MD.
Rieder RO. 2003. Research Training: The Columbia Model. *Psychiatric Research Report* 19(1): 4–7.
Ringel SP, Steiner JF, Vickrey BG, Spencer SS. 2001. Training clinical researchers in neurology: We must do better. *Neurology* 57(3): 388–392.
Roberts LW, Bogenschutz MP. 2001. Preparing the next generation of psychiatric researchers: A story of obstacles and optimism. *Academic Psychiatry* 25(1): 4–7.
Roeske NA. 1976. Women in psychiatry: A review. *American Journal of Psychiatry* 133(4): 365–372.
Rosenberg LE. 1999. The physician-scientist: An essential–and fragile–link in the medical research chain. *Journal of Clinical Investigation* 103(12): 1621–1626.
Rosenberg LE. 2000. Young physician-scientists: Internal medicine's challenge. *Annals of Internal Medicine* 133(10): 831–832.
Rosenberg LE. 2002. Exceptional economic returns on investments in medical research. *Medical Journal of Australia* 177(7): 368–371.
Royall DR, Lauterbach EC, Cummings JL, Reeve A, Rummans TA, Kaufer DI, LaFrance WC, Coffey CE. 2002. Executive control function: A review of its promise and challenges for clinical research. A report from the Committee on Research of the American Neuropsychiatric Association. *Journal of Neuropsychiatry and Clinical Neurosciences* 14(4): 377–405.
Sackett DL, Rosenberg WM, Gray JA, Haynes RB, Richardson WS. 1996. Evidence based medicine: What it is and what it isn't. *British Medical Journal* 312(7023): 71–72.
Scheffler RM, Kirby PB. 2003. The occupational transformation of the mental health system. *Health Affairs* 22(5).
Scheid DC, Hamm RM, Crawford SA. 2002. Measuring academic production. *Family Medicine* 34(1): 34–44.
Schoenbaum M, Unutzer J, Sherbourne C, Duan N, Rubenstein LV, Miranda J, Meredith LS, Carney MF, Wells K. 2001. Cost-effectiveness of practice-initiated quality improvement for depression: Results of a randomized controlled trial. *Journal of the American Medical Association* 286(11): 1325–1330.
Schou M. 1997. Forty years of lithium treatment. *Archives of General Psychiatry* 54(1): 9–15.
Schrier RW. 1997. Ensuring the survival of the clinician-scientist. *Academic Medicine* 72(7): 589–594.
Schwalm DD. 2002a (September 26). *Financial Incentives in Psychiatric Research.* Presentation at the Institute of Medicine Committee on Incorporating Research into Psychiatry Residency Training. Woods Hole, MA.

Schwalm DD. 2002b. *Managed Care and the Incomes of Psychiatrists.* Berkeley, CA: University of California.

SCORE (Service Corps of Retired Executives Association). 2003. *SCORE Homepage.* [Online]. Available: http://www.score.org/ [accessed April 22, 2003].

Shaffer D, Fisher P, Dulcan MK, Davies M, Piacentini J, Schwab-Stone ME, Lahey BB, Bourdon K, Jensen PS, Bird HR, Canino G, Regier DA. 1996. The NIMH diagnostic interview schedule for children version 2.3 (DISC- 2.3): Description, acceptability, prevalence rates, and performance in the MECA study. *Journal of the American Academy of Child and Adolescent Psychiatry* 35(7): 865–877.

Shalala D. 2000. Protecting research subjects–what must be done. *New England Journal of Medicine* 343(11): 808–810.

Shapiro T, Mrazek D, Pincus HA. 1991. Current status of research activity in American child and adolescent psychiatry: Part I. *Journal of the American Academy of Child and Adolescent Psychiatry* 30(3): 443–448.

Sheets KJ, Anderson WA. 1991. The reporting of curriculum development activities in the health professions. *Teaching and Learning in Medicine* 3: 221–226.

Shine KI. 1998. Encouraging clinical research by physician scientists. *Journal of the American Medical Association* 280(16): 1442–1444.

Shore D, Goldschmidts W, Wynne D, Hyman S. 2001. NIMH perspective: Meeting national needs for psychiatrist-researchers. *Academic Psychiatry* 25(1): 9–11.

Sierles FS, Taylor MA. 1995. Decline of U.S. medical student career choice of psychiatry and what to do about it. *American Journal of Psychiatry* 152(10): 1416–1426.

Silverstein SC, Garrison HH, Heinig SJ. 1995. A few basic economic facts about research in the medical and related life sciences. *Policy Forum* 9: 833–840.

Simon JL, Chesney RW, Alden ER, Mulvey HJ, Behrman RE. 2000. The future of pediatric education II: Organizing pediatric education to meet the needs of infants, children, adolescents, and young adults in the 21st century. *Pediatrics* 105(1): 162–212.

Simpson S, Corney R, Fitzgerald P, Beechman J. 2003. A randomized controlled trial to evaluate the effectiveness and cost-effectiveness of psychodynamic counseling for general practice patients with chronic depression. *Psychological Medicine* 33(2): 229–240.

Spar IL, Pryor KC, Simon W. 1993. Effect of debt level on the residency preferences of graduating medical students. *Academic Medicine* 68(7): 570–572.

Steele C, Pincus HA, eds. 1995. *Directory of Research Fellowship Opportunities in Psychiatry.* Washington, DC: APA

Sturm R, Bao Y. 2000. Datapoints: Psychiatric care expenditures and length of stay: Trends in industrialized countries. *Psychiatric Services* 51(3): 295.

Sung NS, Crowley WF, Genel M, Salber P, Sandy L, Sherwood LM, Johnson SB, Catanese V, Tilson H, Getz K, Larson EL, Scheinberg D, Reece EA, Slavkin H, Dobs A, Grebb J, Martinez RA, Korn A, Rimoin D. 2003. Central challenges facing the national clinical research enterprise. *Journal of the American Medical Association* 289(10): 1278–1287.

Sutton J, Killian CD. 1996. The M.D.-Ph.D. researcher: What species of investigator? *Academic Medicine* 71(5): 454–459.

Swartz HA, Cho RY. 2002. Building bridges: The Pittsburgh model of research career development. *Psychiatric Research Report* 18(3): 8–9.

The American Board of Anesthesiology. 2002. *Booklet of Information.* [Online]. Available: http://www.abanes.org/booklet/index.html [accessed April 23, 2003].

The Robert Wood Johnson Foundation. 2001. *National Program Report: Clinical Scholars Program.* [Online]. Available: http://www.rwjf.org/reports/npreports/PROGRAM%20STRUCTURE%20AND%20OPERATIONS [accessed July 18, 2002].

The Robert Wood Johnson Foundation. 2003. *Minority Medical Faculty Development Program.* [Online]. Available: http://www.mmfdp.org/about-.htm [accessed May 8, 2003].

Thornton J, Esposto F. 2003. How important are economic factors in choice of medical specialty? *Health Economics* 12(1): 67–73.

Trinh NH, Hoblyn J, Mohanty S, Yaffe K. 2003. Efficacy of cholinesterase inhibitors in the treatment of neuropsychiatric symptoms and functional impairment in Alzheimer disease: A meta-analysis. *Journal of the American Medical Association* 289(2): 210–216.

Tuma AH, Mitchell W, Brunstetter RW. 1987. Toward a manpower base for research in child psychiatry: Report of three National Institute of Mental Health workshops. *Journal of the American Academy of Child and Adolescent Psychiatry* 26(2): 281–285.

U. S. Census. 2002. *U. S. Census Homepage.* [Online]. Available: http://www-.census.gov [accessed November 14, 2002].

University of Colorado. 2002. *Postdoctoral Research Training Program in Developmental Psychobiology.* [Online]. Available: http://www.uchsc.edu/sm/psych/postdoc/ [accessed May 6, 2003].

University of Connecticut. 2002. *Fellowship Training.* [Online]. Available: http://psychiatry.uchc.edu/training/ [accessed January 22, 2003].

Weston D, Morrison K. 2001. A multidimensional meta-analysis of treatment for depression, panic, and generalized anxiety disorder: An empirical examination of the status of empirically supported therapies. *Journal of Consulting and Clinical Psychology* 69(6): 875–899.

Whelan GP, Gary NE, Kostis J, Boulet JR, Hallock JA. 2002. The changing pool of international medical graduates seeking certification training in U. S. graduate medical education programs. *Journal of the American Medical Association* 288(9): 1079–1084.

Whitcomb ME, Walter DL. 2000. Research training in six selected internal

medicine fellowship programs. *Annals of Internal Medicine* 133(10): 800–807.
White ME, McDonnell SM, Werker DH, Cardenas VM, Thacker SB. 2001. Partnerships in international applied epidemiology training and service, 1975–2001. *American Journal of Epidemiology* 154(11): 993–999.
WHO (World Health Organization). 2001. *The World Health Report 2001. Mental Health: New Understanding, New Hope.* Geneva: WHO
Winstead DK. 2001 (November 7). *ACGME Training Requirements and Research Training in Psychiatry.* National Institute of Mental Health and the American Psychiatric Association Workshop on Research Training for Psychiatrists. Bethesda, MD.
Winstead DK. 2002 (September 26). *ACGME, APBN, and Research Training in Psychiatry: New Directions.* Presentation at the Institute of Medicine Committee on Incorporating Research into Psychiatry Residency Training. Woods Hole, MA.
WPIC (Western Psychiatric Institute and Clinic). 2002a. *Course Descriptions: 5-Year Combined General and Child & Adolescent Psychiatry.* [Online]. Available: http://www.wpic.pitt.edu/education/residency_training/CHLD_COURSES.htm [accessed January 20, 2003].
WPIC. 2002b. *NIMH Undergraduate Fellowship in Mental Health Research.* [Online]. Available: http://www.wpic.pitt.edu/education/ugradmhres/program3.html [accessed March 20, 2003].
WPIC. 2002c. *Residency Training.* [Online]. Available: www.wpic.pitt.edu/education/residency_training [accessed November 12, 2002].
Wyngaarden JB. 1979. The clinical investigator as an endangered species. *New England Journal of Medicine* 301(23): 1254–1259.
Yanai K. 1999. The role of positron emission tomography in neuropharmacology in the living human brain and drug development. *Nippon Yakurigaku Zasshi - Folia Pharmacologica Japonica* 114(3): 169–178.
Zemlo TR, Garrison HH, Partridge NC, Ley TJ. 2000. The physician-scientist: Career issues and challenges at the year 2000. *FASEB Journal* 14(2): 221–230.
Zuvekas SH, Banthin JS, Selden TM. 1998. Mental health parity: What are the gaps in coverage? *Journal of Mental Health Policy and Economics* 3(1): 135–146.

Appendix A

Data Sources and Methods

To respond to the study charge, the committee took several steps to review research training and psychiatry residency training. Sources of data and information included the expertise of the committee members, literature reviews and Internet searches of principal concepts (e.g., research training, program curricula, personal characteristics, funding mechanisms), informal and semistructured interviews, two commissioned works, hosting of a public workshop, and other invited presentations.

STUDY COMMITTEE

The 12-member committee that conducted this study broadly represented psychiatry (adult and child and adolescent psychiatry, from both small and large programs), other biological and cognitive–behavioral disciplines (neurology, psychology, neuroscience), mental health economics, and other branches of medicine (pathology and pediatrics). The committee included members with expertise in either training of biomedical researchers or graduate medical education, biomedical researchers, two psychiatry department chairs, a medical school dean, and a director of a children's hospital research foundation. The committee convened for one 3-day and four 2-day meetings on April 12–13, 2002; June 18–20, 2002; July 30–31, 2002; September 26–27, 2002; and March 17–18, 2003. In addition, a public workshop was held on June 19, 2002. Biographies of individual committee members appear in Appendix D.

LITERATURE REVIEW AND INTERNET SEARCHES

The committee conducted extensive literature reviews and Internet searches regarding research training during residency and factors that either promote or inhibit such activity. In particular, Institute of Medicine (IOM) staff used in-house databases, including Academic Search Premier, PubMed, and PsychInfo, to identify peer-reviewed literature using a combination of the following keywords:

- Psychiatry
- Research
- Residency
- Education
- Graduate medical education
- Research training
- Training
- Internal medicine
- Allergy and immunology
- Neurology
- Pulmonary disease and critical care
- International medical graduates
- Minority physicians
- Women physicians

Furthermore, the committee reviewed residency training requirements and certification requirements for psychiatrists in two ways. First, we reviewed the Accreditation Council for Graduate Medical Education (ACGME) requirements for different specialties, including psychiatry, neurology, internal medicine, and allergy and immunology, to determine key similarities and differences among residency training programs. Second, we reviewed certification requirements established by the American Board of Psychiatry and Neurology (ABPN) for psychiatrists.

INTERVIEWS AND OUTREACH

In addition to the above literature reviews and extensive Internet searches, the committee conducted a number of interviews and outreach activities to understand organizational and individual perspectives as they relate to research training during residency. In an effort to further understand local factors that influence residency-based research training and the factors that influence individual psychiatrists to pursue research, IOM staff conducted outreach in three ways:

- IOM staff interviewed 8 chairs whose departments were considered emerging with respect to interdepartmental research. Chairs were asked a series of questions relating to research activities of residents and faculty, innovative strategies to encourage research within the department, and obstacles to training (see Chapter 4 for further discussion).
- Seven psychiatrist-investigators who had received mentored career (K) awards within the past 5 years (see Chapter 2 for further discussion) were interviewed.
- Members of the American Association of Directors of Psychiatric Residency Training (AADPRT) were solicited via mass mailing to provide programmatic information regarding research programs, as well as data on residents who have tracked to careers in research. Summary information on programmatic characteristics appears in Appendix C, and outcome data on research training efforts at selected institutions appear in Chapter 4.

IOM staff also conducted personal communications with numerous individuals outside of the committee, including but not limited to the following:

- Virginia Anthony, American Academy of Child and Adolescent Psychiatry (May 3, 2002)
- Richard Balon, Wayne State University (March 26, 2003)
- Barbara Barzansky, American Medical Association Council on Medical Education (October 22, 2002)
- James Bentley, American Hospital Association (October 25, 2002)
- Eugene Beresin, Massachusetts General Hospital/McLean Hospital (May 16, 2002)
- Patricia Davidson, American Academy of Child and Adolescent Psychiatry (January 31, 2003)
- Leon Eisenberg, Harvard University (January 30, 2002)
- Karen Fisher, Association of American Medical Colleges Division of Health Care Affairs (July 11, 2002)
- David Folks, University of Nebraska (November 18, 2002)*
- Richard G. Frank, Harvard University; Institute of Medicine Board on Neuroscience and Behavioral Health (March 3, 2003)
- Lawrence Friedman, National Heart, Lung, and Blood Institute, Division of Epidemiology and Clinical Applications (April 17, 2003)
- Gregory Fritz, Brown University (February 10, 2003)
- John C. Gienapp, University of Washington (July 2, 2003)

- J. Christian Gillin, University of California, San Diego (January 8, 2002; February 1, 2002)
- Walter Goldschmidts, National Institute of Mental Health (April 4, 2002; December 12, 2002; February 11, 2003)
- Gary Gottlieb, Brigham and Women's Hospital; Harvard University (June 21, 2002)
- Linda Greco-Sanders, University of Colorado (August 7, 2003)
- John Greden, American Psychiatric Association Council on Research (July 26, 2003)
- Ernesto Guerra, American Psychiatric Association (December 4, 2002; July 15, 2003; July 25, 2003)
- Gretchen Haas, Western Psychiatric Institute and Clinic (April 18, 2003)
- Deborah Hales, American Psychiatric Association (June 13, 2002)
- Jeanne K. Heard, University of Arkansas College of Medicine (June 2003)
- Leighton Huey, University of Connecticut (October 3, 2002)
- Barry Kaplan, National Institutes of Mental Health (July 29, 2002)
- Patricia Kapur, American Board of Anesthesiology (April 15, 2003)
- Martin Keller, Brown University (November 20, 2002)*
- James Leckman, Yale University (April 4, 2003)
- Theodore Marmor, Yale University (August 22, 2002)
- Christopher McDougal, Indiana University (November 4, 2002)*
- Judith G. Miller, National Board of Medical Examiners (July 15, 2003)
- Robert Moore, National Institutes of Health, Office of Reports and Analysis (July 11, 2002)
- David Mrazek, Mayo Clinic (March 24, 2003)
- Henry Nasrallah, Veterans Administration Medical Center (July 29, 2002)
- Charles Nemeroff, Emory University (November 21, 2002)*
- Eric Nestler, University of Texas at Southwestern (November 7, 2002)*
- Jason T. Olin, National Institute of Mental Health, Aging Research Consortium (November 13, 2002)
- John C. Peirce, Good Samaritan Regional Medical Center (June 24, 2003)
- Alicia Permell, National Institute of Mental Health (December 12, 2002)
- Darrel Reiger, American Psychiatric Association (June 7, 2002)
- Mark Rieder, Mayo Clinic (April 10, 2003)
- Ronald Rieder, Columbia University (March 29, 2003)

- Robert Rosencheck, Yale University (August 22, 2002)
- Eugene Rubin, Washington University (May 28, 2002)
- Neal Ryan, Western Psychiatric Institute and Clinic (April 17, 2003)
- Walter Schaffer, National Institutes of Health, Office of Extramural Research (July 11, 2002; September 16, 2003)
- Stephen Scheiber, American Board of Psychiatry and Neurology, (April 5, 2003)
- Bert Shapiro, National Institutes of Health (December 30, 2002)
- Charles Schulz, University of Minnesota (November 22, 2002)*
- Anne L. Shuster, Robert Wood Johnson Clinical Scholars Program (June 12, 2002)
- Joel Silverman, Virginia Commonwealth University (November 5, 2002)*
- G. Richard Smith, Jr., University of Arkansas (December 5, 2002)*
- Cheryl Sroka, Emory University (April 21, 2003)
- Larry Sulton, ACGME (August 6, 2002)
- Fred Taylor, National Institutes of Health, National Center for Research Resources (April 10, 2003)
- G. Warren Teeter, Administrators in Academic Psychiatry (July 19, 2002)
- Linda Thorsen, ACGME (October 15, 2002)
- Glenn Treisman, Johns Hopkins University (May 15, 2002)
- Farris Tuma, National Institute of Mental Health (June 4, 2002)
- Benedetto Vitiello, National Institute of Mental Health, Division of Services and Intervention Research (November 14, 2002)
- Debra F. Weinstein, Massachusetts General Hospital (July 3, 2002)
- Dan Winstead, Tulane University (July 16, 2002)
- Sunny Yoder, Association of American Medical Colleges (June 18, 2003)
- James R. Zaidan, Emory University (June 27, 2003)
- Steven Zalcman, National Institute of Mental Health (April 8, 2002)

* = One of 8 chairs interviewed per outreach noted on page 120.

COMMISSIONED PAPERS

The committee commissioned the work of historian Joel T. Braslow of the University of California at Los Angeles and economist Douglas D.

Schwalm of Louisiana State University. Braslow was commissioned to write a paper considering the unique history of psychiatric practice and how that history influenced the emergence of research activity within the field. The paper focuses on the late twentieth century. Braslow's work was important for the preparation of the section on pscyhodynamics that appears in Chapter 3. Schwalm used data from the American Psychiatric Association to consider the income differences that exist between psychiatrists who are and are not engaged in research activity. Schwalm's analysis additionally controlled for gender, race, practice venue, and experience. Schwalm's results are cited and used throughout the report, especially in Chapter 5.

PUBLIC WORKSHOP

As noted above, the committee convened for five 2-day meetings and a separate 1-day public workshop. The workshop focused on obstacles to research training in psychiatry. Most of the invited speakers were experts in adult or child and adolescent psychiatry, although experts in economics, neurology, and clinical research also presented their views. A list of speakers and participants who attended the open sessions of the committee meetings and the workshop is presented below.

Open Session for Committee Meeting #1
April 12–13, 2002
The National Academies
Washington, DC

1:00 p.m.–2:15 p.m.	**Sponsor Presentation of Study Genesis and Charge** Richard K. Nakamura, *Acting Director, National Institute of Mental Health* Wayne S. Fenton, *Acting Deputy Director, National Institute of Mental Health*
2:15 p.m.–3:15 p.m.	**The Psychiatry Residency Paths** Sheldon I. Miller, *Chair, Psychiatry Department, Northwestern University; Past Chair, Psychiatry Residency Review Committee*
3:30 p.m.–4:15 p.m.	**The Internal Medicine and Allergy and Immunology Residency Paths** Stephen I. Wasserman, *Professor of Medicine, University of California at San Diego; Past Chair, American Board of Allergy and Immunology*

Open Session for Committee Meeting #2
Tuesday, June 18, 2002
The National Academies
Washington, DC

10:00 a.m.–10:50 a.m.	**Obstacles to Residency-based Research Training in Psychiatry** Herbert Pardes, M.D., *President and CEO, New York-Presbyterian Hospital; Former Director, National Institute of Mental Health*
11:30 a.m.–12:20 p.m.	**Obstacles to Residency-based Research Training in Psychiatry** Steven E. Hyman, M.D., *Provost, Harvard University; Former Director, National Institute of Mental Health*
4:00 p.m.–4:50 p.m.	**Obstacles to Residency-based Research Training in Psychiatry** Harold A. Pincus, M.D., *Professor and Executive Vice-Chairman, Department of Psychiatry, University of Pittsburgh, School of Medicine, Western Psychiatric Institute and Clinic; Senior Scientist and Director, RAND–University of Pittsburgh Health Institute*

Open Session for Committee Meeting #3
July 30–31, 2002
The National Academies
Washington, DC

1:00 p.m.–2:00 p.m. **Review of Strategies Used by Pediatrics**
James A. Stockman III, M.D., President, American Board of Pediatrics

Open Session for Committee Meeting #4
September 26–27 2002
J. Erik Jonsson Center
Woods Hole, Massachusetts

9:00 a.m.–10:00 a.m. **Daniel K. Winstead, M.D.**
Chair, Department of Psychiatry and Neurology, Tulane University Health Sciences Center; Chair, Psychiatry Residency Review Committee; ACGME President; American Association of Chairs in Psychiatry

10:15 a.m.–11:15 a.m. **Joel T. Braslow, M.D., Ph.D.**
Associate Professor, Departments of Psychiatry and Biobehavioral Sciences and History, University of California at Los Angeles

Invited Discussant: Gerald N. Grob, Ph.D.
Henry E. Sigerist Professor of History of Medicine Emeritus, Rutgers University

11:15 a.m.–12:00 p.m. **Douglas D. Schwalm, Ph.D.**
Assistant Professor, Department of Economics, Louisiana State University

Public Workshop on Obstacles to the Incorporation of Research into Psychiatry Residency Training
Wednesday, June 19, 2002
The National Academies
Washington, DC

8:30 a.m.–8:50 a.m. **Ensuring the Future of Clinical Research Across Medical Specialties**
Roger E. Meyer, M.D., Senior Consultant for Clinical Research, Association of American Medical Colleges

8:50 a.m.–9:10 a.m. Questions and Discussion

9:10 a.m.–9:30 a.m.	**Personal Economics and Other Factors Influencing Specialty Selection** *Sean M. Nicholson, Ph.D., Assistant Professor of Health Care Systems, The Wharton School of the University of Pennsylvania*
9:30 a.m.–9:50 a.m.	Questions and Discussion
10:05 a.m.–10:25 a.m.	**Mentoring Residents Interested in Research** *James H. Meador-Woodruff, M.D., Associate Chair for Research Training and Faculty Development, Department of Psychiatry, and Senior Associate Research Scientist, Mental Health Research Institute, University of Michigan*
10:25 a.m.–10:45 a.m.	Questions and Discussion
10:45 a.m.–11:00 a.m.	**Child Psychiatry's Perspective, Part I** *David Shaffer, F.R.C.P., F.R.C.Psych., Director of Child Psychiatry, Columbia University, New York State Psychiatric Institute*
11:00 a.m.–11:15 a.m.	**Child Psychiatry's Perspective, Part II** *John S. March, M.D., Director of Programs in Child and Adolescent Anxiety Disorders and Developmental Psychopharmacology, Duke University*
11:15 a.m.–11:35 a.m.	Questions and Discussion
12:35 p.m.–12:50 p.m.	**Leadership Perspectives: From the Executive's Perch** *Steven M. Mirin, M.D., Medical Director, American Psychiatric Association; Former President and Psychiatrist-in-Chief, McLean Hospital*
12:50 p.m.–1:05 p.m.	**Leadership Perspectives: Where the Chair Sits, Part I** *Paula J. Clayton, M.D., Professor of Psychiatry, University of New Mexico; Professor Emeritus of Psychiatry and Former Chair, Department of Psychiatry, University of Minnesota*
1:05 p.m.–1:20 p.m.	**Leadership Perspectives: Where the Chair Sits, Part II** *Henry A. Nasrallah, M.D., Professor of Psychiatry, Neurology and Internal Medicine, University*

	of Mississippi School of Medicine, and Chief, Mental Health Services, VA Medical Center, Jackson, Mississippi; Former Chair, Department of Psychiatry, Ohio State University
1:20 p.m.–1:40 p.m.	Questions and Discussion
1:40 p.m.–2:00 p.m.	**Recruitment, Development, and Retention of Clinical Neuroscientists in Residency Training: Neurology's Perspective** Robert C. Griggs, M.D., Chair of Neurology, University of Rochester; Editor-in-Chief, Neurology
2:00 p.m.–2:20 p.m.	Questions and Discussion
2:20 p.m.–2:35 p.m.	**Sociocultural and Policy Issues in Psychiatry Residency Training** Howard H. Goldman, M.D., Ph.D., Director of Mental Health Policy Studies, University of Maryland, Baltimore
2:35 p.m.–2:50 p.m.	Questions and Discussion
3:05 p.m.–4:05 p.m.	**Reflections/Comments from Current and Former Training Directors** Martin J. Drell, M.D., Louisiana State University Christopher R. Thomas, M.D., The University of Texas Medical Branch at Galveston Karon Dawkins, M.D., University of North Carolina, Chapel Hill Lisa B. Dixon, M.D., Department of Psychiatry, University of Maryland, Baltimore Anthony L. Rostain, M.D., University of Pennsylvania

Appendix B

Federal and Other Funding Mechanisms Listed and Summarized by Career Stage

The following table describes funding sources for mental health research that are available to undergraduate students, medical students, residents, fellows, junior faculty, and institutions that train individuals across this entire educational spectrum. Federal and other sources of funding are listed.

Federal and Other Funding Mechanisms Listed and Summarized by Career Stage

Grant Title	Funding Agency	Duration	Magnitude	Description
Undergraduate				
Summer Internship Program in Biomedical Research[1]	NIH	>8 weeks	Stipend: ≤$2,400/month	Interns work at a designated NIH-funded research laboratory. Also available to graduate students.
Mental Health Research Education Grant (R25)[2]	NIH/NIMH	1–5 years	<$250,000/year in direct costs with indirect costs of 8%; 3–5 grants awarded each year	Funds educational programs for all levels of mental health researchers, including residents.
Scholars Program[3]	Stanley Medical Research Institute	6–8 weeks	>$15,000/year; supported 174 students in 2001	Began in 1989. Provides research exposure to undergraduates and medical students.
Medical School				
Research Fellowship Program[4]	NIH	>10 weeks	≤$2,500/month; 80–90 selected each year	First- through third-year graduate students work at NIH-cooperating institutions and attend grand rounds, lectures, and seminars. ~30% success rate.

Medical Scientist Training Program (MSTP)[5]	NIH/NIGMS	7–8 years	NRSA stipend; full tuition; institution allowance, <$6,000; funded 38 programs and 890 positions in 1999	Began in 1964. Provides combined M.D./Ph.D. degree. Outcome data show that graduates are more likely than M.D. graduates to have research support, hold academic positions, and apply for and receive NIH grants.
Ruth L. Kirschstein NRSA Predoctoral M.D./Ph.D. Fellowship (F30)[6]	NIH/NIMH	6 years	Stipend: $20,000; ≥60% of tuition; institution allowance: <$2,750	Provides intense research training.
Ruth L. Kirschstein NRSA Predoctoral Fellowship (F31)[7]	NIH/NIMH	5 years	Stipend: $20,000; ≥60% of tuition; institution allowance: <$2,750; NIH funded 200–400 applications annually from 1990 to 2001	Special eligibility for racial and ethnic minorities and individuals with disabilities.
Clinical Elective Program[8]	NIMH	6–8 weeks	Travel and rent subsidy: $300	Tutorial program for medical students who have completed psychiatry rotation.

Continued

Federal and Other Funding Mechanisms Listed and Summarized by Career Stage

Grant Title	Funding Agency	Duration	Magnitude	Description
Clinical Research Fellowship Program[9]	Doris Duke Charitable Foundation	1 year	$20,000 plus health insurance	Began in 2000. Available for third-year medical students who take a year out to participate in the program. Ten medical schools are selected for participation and can nominate at least 5 applicants.
Residency				
PGY4 Residency Training[10]	NIMH	1 year	Stipend: $46,000; infrastructure support: $2,500; supported 6 adult and 2 child psychiatrists in 2002	Available to outstanding PGY4 residents. Involvement in clinical research at state-of-the-art Magnuson Center.
Jeanne Spurlock Research Fellowship in Drug Abuse and Addiction for Minority Medical Students[11]	AACAP and NIDA	Summer (12 weeks)	Stipend: $2,500; travel to AACAP meeting; 5 slots available	Available for racial minority residents to conduct mentored research.

Jeanne Spurlock Minority Medical Student Clinical Fellowship in Child and Adolescent Psychiatry[12]	AACAP	Summer (12 weeks)	Stipend: $2,500; travel to AACAP meeting; 14 slots available	Available for racial minority residents to conduct mentored research.
Health Services Research Scholars Program[13]	APIRE and GlaxoSmithKline		$7,000; 5 slots available	Available to residents, fellows, and junior faculty to analyze data on mental health care costs and utilization. Funding available for mentoring and travel.
Scholars in Research on Severe Mental Illness[14]	APIRE and Janssen Pharmaceuticals	2 years	$5,000; travel to APA meeting	Available to PGY1 to PGY3 residents interested in mental health research careers.
Travel Grants[15]	AACAP and Pfizer Pharmaceuticals	6-day meeting	$800 to travel to AACAP meeting; 50 awards available for child and adolescent psychiatrists	Individual institutions receive award and select residents.
General Resident Fellows Program[16]	AACAP and Eli Lilly	6-day meeting	$1,500 to travel to AACAP meeting; 20 awards available for adult (general) psychiatrists	Individual institutions receive award and select residents.

Continued

Federal and Other Funding Mechanisms Listed and Summarized by Career Stage

Grant Title	Funding Agency	Duration	Magnitude	Description
Presidential Scholar Award[17]	AACAP and Bristol-Myers Squibb	1 week	$2,500 for travel to mentoring site and to AACAP meeting; 5 slots available	Available to child and adolescent psychiatry residents interested in research and public policy.
Research Colloquium for Junior Investigators[18]	APIRE and NIH institutes (NIAAA, NIDA, and NIMH)	All-day workshop	$1,000 for travel expenses; 45 awards available	Began in 1996. Program guides and encourages senior residents, fellows, and junior faculty.
Fellowship				
Clinical Research Curriculum Award (K30)[19]	NIH (administered by NHLBI)	5 years	$200,000/year; funded 59 grants for $12 million in 2002	Supports creation or improvement of clinical research curriculum aimed at clinically trained individuals.
Ruth L. Kirschstein NRSA Institutional Research Training Grant (T32)[20]	NIH	3–5 years	Stipend: ≤$51,000; ≥60% of tuition; institution allowance: <$6,000; funded 1,000 for $134 million in 2002	Grant supports teaching and training of undergraduates, graduate students, residents (in limited circumstances), and fellows. Success rate in 2002 across NIH was 58%.

217

Ruth L. Kirschstein NRSA for Individual Postdoctoral Fellows (F32)[21]	NIH	3 years	Stipend: ≤$51,000; ≥60% of tuition; institution allowance: <$6,000; NIH funded 614 grants for ~$26 million in 2002	Began in 1974. Supports independent investigators to broaden research backgrounds. Success rate in 2002 was 40%.
Clinical Associates Program (Psychiatry)[22]	NIMH	2 years	Stipend: ≤$64,000, institutional support: $2,500; 6–13 slots available each year	Program exposes fellows to clinical and basic research and focuses on clinical care of research subjects, research protocol development, and preparation of study results.
M.D./Ph.D. Psychiatry Research Fellowship[23]	APIRE and Wyeth Pharmaceuticals	1 year	Stipend: $45,000; 2 slots available/year	Fellows are required to spend 85% effort on research activities.
Severe Mental Illness Research Fellowship[24]	APIRE and GlaxoSmithKline	1 year	Stipend: $45,000; 2 slots available/year	Fellows are required to spend 85% effort on research training in severe mental illness. Institution may augment stipend if desired.
Psychiatric Research Fellowship[25]	APIRE and Eli Lilly	1 year	Stipend: $45,000; 2 slots available	Began 1988. Supports postresidency psychiatrists who conduct research at 85% effort. Institution may augment stipend.

Continued

Federal and Other Funding Mechanisms Listed and Summarized by Career Stage

Grant Title	Funding Agency	Duration	Magnitude	Description
Klingenstein Third Generation Fellowship[26]	Esther A. and Joseph Klingenstein Fund	2 years	Stipend: $30,000; 2–4 fellows selected each year	Program provides support to study child and adolescent depression prior to applying for NIMH grant. Outcome data for 1998 to 2004 on 12 graduates: 8 are principal investigators on NIMH K or R awards; 5 have received NARSAD Young Investigator Awards. In total, they have published 48 articles, 33 abstracts, and 9 book chapters.
Young Investigator Award Program[27]	NARSAD	1–2 years	Stipend: $30,000; 175 awards in 2003.	Began in 1987. Program funds research in serious mental illness, including schizophrenia and major affective disorders.
Clinical Scholars Program[28]	The Robert Wood Johnson Foundation	2 years	Stipend: $44,000; 905 scholars funded from 1973 through 2000	Began in 1973. Program trains young scientists in nonbiological disciplines important to medical care systems. Seven participating institutions offer these fellowships. Most graduates have entered academic medicine.

Fellowship in Clinical Neuropsychopharmacology[29]	ACNP and GlaxoSmithKline	1 year	Stipend: $45,000; institution: $10,000; travel to ACNP annual meetings	Program seeks to increase the number of investigators in clinical neuropsychopharmacology. For fellows and junior faculty.
Young Investigator Award[30]	Borderline Personality Disorder Research Foundation	2 years	$75,000; 11 selected in 2003	Began in 2003. Program supports clinical and basic research.
Markey Scholars Award[31]	Markey Foundation	7–8 years (2 years as fellow, 5 years as faculty)	Stipend: $15,000+; institution: $200,000 over 5 years; 16 recipients selected annually	From 1983 to 1997, 113 scholars conducted basic biomedical research as they transitioned from fellows to junior faculty members.
Career Award in the Biomedical Sciences Program[32]	Burroughs Wellcome Fund	5 years; 14–26 selected annually	$500,000 over 5 years	Began in 1994. Program funds postdoctoral training and 3 years as faculty member to conduct biomedical research at 80% time. From 1995 to 1999, 77% obtained a faculty position, and 78% were principal investigators on one or more grants (mainly from NIH).

Continued

219

Federal and Other Funding Mechanisms Listed and Summarized by Career Stage

Grant Title	Funding Agency	Duration	Magnitude	Description
Early Faculty Career				
Mentored Research Scientist Development Award (K01)[33]	NIH/NIMH	3–5 years	Stipend: $90,000; infrastructure: $50,000; NIMH funded 124 grants at a cost of $15.7 million in 2002	Grant requires 75% effort.
Mentored Clinical Scientist Development Award (K08)[34]	NIMH	3–5 years	Stipend: $90,000; infrastructure: $50,000; NIMH funded 93 grants at a cost of $14 million in 2002	Grant requires 75% effort. Provides mentored research experiences for individuals seeking to become clinical researchers, and integrates didactic with lab/field research.
Behavioral Science Track Award for Rapid Transition (B/START)[35]	NIMH	1 year	$50,000; NIMH funded 266 grants from 1994 to 2001; 20–55 applicants are funded each year	Funds available for research projects related to behavioral science. Applicants must have no more than 5 years postdoctoral experience.

Small Grants (R03)[36]	NIMH	1–2 years	$50,000/year in direct costs	Funds exploratory studies or efforts to develop new methods or techniques.
Exploratory/Development Grant Program (R21)[37]	NIMH	2 years	$275,000 over 2 years	Topics include pilot effectiveness trials for mental disorders, therapeutic effectiveness protocol development, mental health intervention research, and adherence to interventions for mental disorders.
First Independent Research Support and Transition Award (R29)[38]	NIMH	5 years	$350,000 for 5 years	Discontinued in 1998. Program provided awardees with skills to apply for future grants.
NIMH Research Career Award for Transition to Independence (K22)[39]	NIMH	5 years (3 intramural, 2 extramural)	Intramural phase: $140,000/year in direct costs (stipend: $90,000); NIH funded 92 grants at $13 million in 2002	Provides research training (both at NIMH and at an extramural institution) for postdoctorates with 2–5 years of training. Trainees are required to give 75% effort to research in the extramural phase.

Continued

Federal and Other Funding Mechanisms Listed and Summarized by Career Stage

Grant Title	Funding Agency	Duration	Magnitude	Description
Mentored Patient-Oriented Research Career Development Award (K23)[40]	NIH	3–5 years	Stipend: $90,000; infrastructure: $50,000; NIMH funded 98 grants at a cost of $15 million in 2002	Began in 1998. Award requires 75% effort. A survey of K23 awardees indicates that it is good preparation for an R01, but that clinical time and funding for expenses and administrative costs are limited.
Young Faculty Award for Research Development in Biological Psychiatry[41]	APIRE and GlaxoSmithKline		Stipend: $45,000	Supports research on mood disorders and/or anxiety disorders.
Elaine Schlosser Lewis Pilot Research Award for Attention Disorders[42]	AACAP and Eli Lilly	1 year	$9,000	Award given to those with full-time academic appointments, less than 2 years of postgraduate experience, and a focus on research on attention disorders.
Travel Fellowship[43]	Bristol-Myers Squibb and ACNP	1 week	Travel funds; 12 fellowships awarded in 2002	For Ph.D. with less than 5 years of postgraduate experience or M.D. with less than 10–12 years of postgraduate experience.

Institutional Support

Centers of Biomedical Research Excellence (COBRE)[44]	NCRR/NIH	5 years	$1.5 million/year (with $500,000 one-time additional support); 15 institutions funded in 2002; state can submit no more than 3 applications	Provides infrastructure support to states that historically have received low NIH support.
Biomedical Research Infrastructure Network (BRIN)[45]	NCRR/NIH	3 years	$2 million/year; state cannot submit more than 2 applications	Began in 1993. Provided for institutions to build research infrastructure in 23 states that have accounted for only 8% of research grants awarded by the NIH in 1998.
Research Project Grant (R01)[46]	NIMH/NIH	2–5 years	Varies (requests for direct costs of >$500,000/year require prior approval from institute)	Investigator-initiated or investigator response to specific research areas (e.g., NIMH has award for studies on mental disorders and AIDS). NIMH awarded 420 grants at a cost of $151 million in 2002.

Continued

Federal and Other Funding Mechanisms Listed and Summarized by Career Stage

Grant Title	Funding Agency	Duration	Magnitude	Description
Minority Research Infrastructure Support Program (M-RISP) (R24)[47]	NIMH	3–5 years	$400,000/year in direct costs	Supports both institutional research development and individual investigator research projects. Institutions must have significant enrollment (>30%) of minority students or must collaborate with a Native American tribe.

NOTES: AACAP = American Academy of Child and Adolescent Psychiatry; ACNP = American College of Neuropsychopharmacology; APIRE = American Psychiatric Institute for Research and Education; NARSAD = National Alliance for Research on Schizophrenia and Depression; NCRR = National Center for Research Resources; NHLBI = National Heart, Lung, and Blood Institute; NIAAA = National Institute on Alcohol Abuse and Alcoholism; NIDA = National Institute on Drug Abuse; NIGMS = National Institute of General Medical Services; NIH = National Institutes of Health; NIMH = National Institute of Mental Health; and NRSA = National Research Service Award

SOURCES:
[1] *Summer Internship Program in Biomedical Research Catalog.* [Online]. Available: http://www.training.nih.gov/student/sip/catalog/program.asp [accessed May 6, 2003].
[2] *Mental Health Research Education Grants (PAR-02-087).* [Online]. Available: http://grants2.nih.gov/grants/guide/pa-files/PAR-02-087.html [accessed May 6, 2003].
[3] *Stanley Scholars Program.* [Online]. Available: http://www.stanleyresearch.org/programs/stanley_scholars.asp [accessed May 6, 2003]; Personal communication, K. Wilson, Stanley Medical Research Institute, December 9, 2002.
[4] *Summer Research Fellowship Program Catalog.* [Online]. Available: http://www.training.nih.gov/student/srfp/catalog/index.asp [accessed May 6, 2003]; *Frequently Asked Questions.* [Online]. Available: http://www.training.nih.gov/student/srfp/faq.asp [accessed May 6, 2003].
[5] *The Careers and Professional Activities of Graduates of the NIGMS Medical Scientist Training Program, September 1998.* [Online]. Available: http://www.nigms.nih.gov/news/reports/mstpstudy/mstp-print.html#summary [accessed May 6, 2003]; AAMC (Association of American Medical Colleges).

SOURCES Continued (Federal and Other Funding Mechanisms Listed and Summarized by Career Stage):

1999. *For the Health of the Public: Ensuring the Future of Clinical Research.* Washington, DC: AAMC; *Training and Career Grant Mechanisms.* [Online]. Available: http://www.nigms.nih.gov/funding/ee [accessed May 6, 2003].

[6] *Individual Predoctoral National Research Service Awards for M.D./Ph.D. Fellowships.* [Online]. Available: http://grants.nih.gov/grants/guide/pa-files/PA-99-089.html [accessed May 6, 2003]; *NIMH Fellowship Information.* [Online]. Available: http://www.nimh.nih.gov/grants/Fellowship1.pdf [accessed May 8, 2003].

[7] *National Research Service Awards for Individual Predoctoral Fellows.* [Online]. Available: http://grants1.nih.gov/grants/guide/pa-files/PA-00-125.html [accessed May 6, 2003]; *NIH Predoctoral Fellowship Award for Minority Students (F31).* [Online]. Available: http://grants1.nih.gov/grants/guide/pa-files/PA-00-069.html [accessed May 6, 2003]; *NIH Predoctoral Fellowship Awards for Students with Disabilities (F31).* [Online]. Available: http://grants.nih.gov/grants/guide/pa-files/PA-00-068.html [accessed May 6, 2003]; *Number of Fellowship (F31) Applications Reviewed and Awarded, Fiscal Years 1990–2001.* [Online]. Available: http://grants1.nih.gov/grants/training/data/tf_trends/sld014.htm [accessed May 6, 2003]; *NIMH Fellowship Information.* [Online]. Available: http://www.nimh.nih.gov/grants/Fellowship1.pdf [accessed May 8, 2003].

[8] *Clinical Electives Program.* [Online]. Available: http://intramural.nimh.nih.gov/training/cep.htm [accessed May 6, 2003]; *Research and Training Opportunities at the National Institutes of Health – Clinical Electives Program.* [Online]. Available: http://www.training.nih.gov/student/cep/index.asp [accessed May 6, 2003].

[9] *Doris Duke Clinical Research Fellowship Program for Medical Students.* [Online]. Available: http://ddcf.aibs.org/crf2000/index.asp [accessed May 6, 2003].

[10] *PGY4 Residency Training Program.* [Online]. Available: http://intramural.nimh.nih.gov/training/pgy4.htm [accessed May 6, 2003]; *PGY-4 Psychiatric Residency Program.* [Online]. Available: http://intramural.nimh.nih.gov/training/pgy4-programexp.pdf [accessed May 6, 2003]; Personal communication, B. Kaplan, NIMH, July 29, 2002.

[11] *Jeanne Spurlock Research Fellowship in Drug Abuse and Addiction for Minority Medical Students.* [Online]. Available: http://www.aacap.org/research/Spurlck1.htm [accessed May 6, 2003]; *Summer Fellowship Application Jeanne Spurlock Research Fellowship in Drug Abuse and Addiction for Minority Medical Students.* [Online]. Available: http://www.aacap.org/awards/2003/sda.pdf [accessed May 6, 2003].

[12] *Jeanne Spurlock Minority Medical Student Clinical Fellowship in Child and Adolescent Psychiatry.* [Online]. Available: http://www.aacap.org/research/Spurlck2.htm [accessed May 6, 2003]; *Summer Fellowship Application Jeanne Spurlock Minority Medical Student Clinical Fellowship in Child and Adolescent Psychiatry.* [Online]. Available: http://www.aacap.org/awards/2003/cfcap.pdf [accessed May 6, 2003].

SOURCES Continued (Federal and Other Funding Mechanisms Listed and Summarized by Career Stage):

[13] American Psychiatric Institute for Research and Education/GlaxoSmithKline 2003 Health Services Research Scholars Program Request for Proposals. [Online]. Available: http://www.psychiatry.org/res_res/Health_Services.cfm [accessed May 6, 2003].
[14] American Psychiatric Institute for Research and Education/Janssen Scholars in Research on Severe Mental Illness. [Online]. Available: http://www.psych.org/res_res/janssen.cfm [accessed May 6, 2003].
[15] AACAP Travel Grant Award. [Online]. Available: http://www.aacap.org/awards/pfizerTravel.htm [accessed May 6, 2003].
[16] AACAP Travel Grant Award. [Online]. Available: http://www.aacap.org/awards/lillyTravel.htm [accessed May 6, 2003].
[17] Presidential Scholar Award. [Online]. Available: http://www.aacap.org/awards/pres.htm [accessed May 6, 2003].
[18] Request for Nominations APA's Research Colloquium for Junior Investigators. [Online]. Available: http://www.psych.org/res_res/03colloquium1903.doc [accessed May 6, 2003]; Personal communication, E. Guerra, American Psychiatric Association, June 19, 2002.
[19] Clinical Research Curriculum Award. [Online]. Available: http://grants2.nih.gov/grants/guide/rfa-files/RFA-OD-00-002.html [accessed May 6, 2003]; NIH Research Training Opportunities: K30 Clinical Research Curriculum Award. [Online]. Available: http://grants1.nih.gov/training/k30.htm [accessed May 6, 2003]; NIH Career Development Awards, Fiscal Year 2002. [Online]. Available: http://grants1.nih.gov/grants/award/training/careerdev02.htm [accessed May 6, 2003].
[20] NIH National Research Service Award Institutional Research Training Grants (T32). [Online]. Available: http://grants1.nih.gov/grants/guide/pa-files/PA-02-109.html [accessed May 6, 2003]; NRSA Stipend Increase and Other Budgetary Changes Effective for Fiscal Year 2002. [Online]. Available: http://grants1.nih.gov/grants/guide/notice-files/NOT-OD-02-028.html [accessed May 6, 2003]; NIH Competing Applications for F32 and T32 Awards, Fiscal Year 1996–2002. [Online]. Available: http://grants1.nih.gov/grants/award/training/f32t329602.htm [accessed May 6, 2003].
[21] National Research Service Awards for Individual Postdoctoral Fellows (F32). [Online]. Available: http://grants1.nih.gov/grants/guide/pa-files/PA-00-104.html [accessed May 6, 2003]; Ruth L. Kirschstein National Research Service Awards for Individual Postdoctoral Fellows (F32). [Online]. Available: http://grants1.nih.gov/grants/guide/pa-files/PA-03-067.html [accessed May 6, 2003]; Number of Fellowship (F32) Applications Reviewed and Awarded Fiscal Years 1990–2001. [Online]. Available: http://grants1.nih.gov/training/data/tf_trends/sld015.htm [accessed May 6, 2003]; NIH Competing Applications for F32 and T32 Awards, Fiscal Year 1996–2002. [Online]. Available: http://grants1.nih.gov/grants/award/training/f32t329602.htm [accessed May 6, 2003]; NIMH Fellowship Information. [Online]. Available: http://www.nimh.nih.gov/grants/Fellowship1.pdf [accessed May 8, 2003].

SOURCES Continued (Federal and Other Funding Mechanisms Listed and Summarized by Career Stage):

[22] *NIMH Clinical Associates Program.* [Online]. Available: http://intramural.nimh.nih.gov/training/cap.htm [accessed May 6, 2003]; *Training Programs for Physicians – Psychiatry.* [Online]. Available: http://www.training.nih.gov/clinical/physician/asp/index.asp [accessed May 6, 2003]; Personal communication, B. Kaplan, NIH, July 29, 2002.
[23] *APIRE/Wyeth Pharmaceuticals M.D./Ph.D. Psychiatric Research Fellowship.* [Online]. Available: http://www.psych.org/res_res/wyeth.cfm [accessed May 6, 2003].
[24] *APIRE/GlaxoSmithKline Severe Mental Illness Psychiatric Research Fellowship.* [Online]. Available: http://www.psych.org/res_res/gskmental_illness.cfm [accessed May 6, 2003].
[25] *Application Guidelines for the APIRE/Lilly Psychiatric Research Fellowship.* [Online]. Available: http://www.psych.org/res_res/lilly.cfm [accessed May 6, 2003].
[26] *Fellowships.* [Online]. Available: http://www.ktgf.org/fellow.html [accessed May 6, 2003]; Personal communication, Y. Moore, Klingenstein Third Generation Foundation, December 6, 2002.
[27] *NARSAD's Young Investigator Award.* [Online]. Available: http://www.narsad.org/research/yiprogram.html [accessed May 6, 2003]; *Year 2004 Guidelines NARSAD's Young Investigator Award.* [Online]. Available: http://www.narsad.org/research/yigdlns.html [accessed May 6, 2003].
[28] *Call for Applications: The Robert Wood Johnson Clinical Scholars Program 2003.* [Online]. Available: http://www.uams.edu/rwjcsp/ [accessed May 6, 2003]; *Clinical Scholars Program.* [Online]. Available: http://www.rwjf.org/reports/npreports/PROGRAM%20STRUCTURE%20AND%20OPERATIONS [accessed May 6, 2003]; AAMC. 1999. *For the Health of the Public: Ensuring the Future of Clinical Research.* Washington, DC: AAMC.
[29] *2003 GlaxoSmithKline Fellowship in Clinical Neuropsychopharmacology.* [Online]. Available: http://www.acnp.org/fellowship.php [accessed May 6, 2003].
[30] *2003 Awards.* [Online]. Available: http://www.borderlineresearch.org/guidelines/index.html [accessed May 6, 2003]; *BPDRF Young Investigator Award 2003 Guidelines.* [Online]. Available: http://www.borderlineresearch.org/guidelines/bpdrf_young_investigator_guidelines.pdf [accessed May 5, 2003].
[31] King J. 1989. Lucille Markey trust sets agenda for going out of business. *The Scientist* 3(10):17; NRC (National Research Council). 1994. *The Funding of Young Investigators in the Biological and Biomedical Sciences.* Washington, DC: National Academy Press; Pion G, Ionescu-Pioggia M. 2003. Bridging postdoctoral training and a faculty position: Initial outcomes of the Burroughs Wellcome Fund Career Awards in the biomedical sciences. *Academic Medicine* 78 (2):177–185

SOURCES Continued (Federal and Other Funding Mechanisms Listed and Summarized by Career Stage):

[32] Pion G, Ionescu-Pioggia M. 2003. Bridging postdoctoral training and a faculty position: Initial outcomes of the Burroughs Wellcome Fund Career Awards in the biomedical sciences. *Academic Medicine* 78(2):177–185.

[33] *NIMH Policy Update for Career Awards (K-Series)*. [Online]. Available: http://grants.nih.gov/grants/guide/notice-files/NOT-MH-02-001.html [accessed May 6, 2003]; *Mentored Research Scientist Development Award – Individual Award (K01)*. [Online]. Available: http://grants2.nih.gov/training/careerdev/mentoredresearchk01 [accessed May 6, 2003]; *Trends in K Applications and Awards—FY 1994–FY 2001*. [Online]. Available: http://grants1.nih.gov/training/data/K_FY2001/index.htm [accessed May 6, 2003]; *NIH Career Development Awards, Fiscal Year 2002*. [Online]. Available: http://grants1.nih.gov/grants/award/training/careerdev02.htm [accessed May 6, 2003].

[34] *Mentored Clinical Scientist Development Award (K08)*. [Online]. Available: http://grants.nih.gov/grants/guide/pa-files/PA-00-003.html [accessed May 6, 2003]; *NIMH Policy Update for Career Awards (K-Series)*. [Online]. Available: http://grants.nih.gov/grants/guide/notice-files/NOT-MH-02-001.html [accessed May 6, 2003]; *NIH Career Development Awards, Fiscal Year 2002*. [Online]. Available: http://grants1.nih.gov/grants/award/training/careerdev02.htm [accessed May 6, 2003].

[35] *Behavioral Science Track Award for Rapid Transition (B/START)*. [Online]. Available: http://grants1.nih.gov/grants/guide/pa-files/PAR-00-119.html [accessed May 6, 2003]; *Application Instructions for Revised Behavioral Science Track Award for Rapid Transition (B/START) Applications (Addendum to PAR-00-119)*. [Online]. Available: http://grants1.nih.gov/grants/guide/notice-files/NOT-MH-01-004.html [accessed May 6, 2003]; Chernoff NN. 2002. NIMH B/START grants are starting blocks for new PIs. *APS Observer* 15(8):1–19.

[36] *NIMH Small Grants Program*. [Online]. Available: http://grants1.nih.gov/grants/guide/pa-files/PAR-99-140.html [accessed May 6, 2003]; *NIMH Small Grants Program*. [Online]. Available: http://grants1.nih.gov/grants/guide/pa-files/PA-03-039.html [accessed May 6, 2003].

[37] *NIH Exploratory/Developmental Research Grant Award (R21)*. [Online]. Available: http://grants1.nih.gov/grants/guide/pa-files/PA-03-107.html [accessed May 6, 2003].

[38] *PA for First Independent Research Support and Transition (FIRST) Award*. [Online]. Available: http://www.nimh.nih.gov/research/first.cfm [accessed May 6, 2003].

[39] *NIMH Research Career Award for Transition to Independence*. [Online]. Available: http://grants1.nih.gov/grants/guide/pa-files/PAR-01-065.html [accessed May 6, 2003]; *NIMH Policy Update for Career Awards (K-Series)*. [Online]. Available: http://grants.nih.gov/grants/guide/notice-files/NOT-MH-02-001.html [accessed May 6, 2003]; *NIH Career Development Awards, Fiscal Year 2002*. [Online]. Available: http://grants1.nih.gov/grants/award/training/careerdev02.htm [accessed May 6, 2003].

SOURCES Continued (Federal and Other Funding Mechanisms Listed and Summarized by Career Stage):

[40] *Mentored Patient-Oriented Research Career Development Award (K23).* [Online]. Available: http://grants1.nih.gov/grants/guide/pa-files/PA-00-004.html [accessed May 6, 2003]; *NIMH Policy Update for Career Awards (K-Series).* [Online]. Available: http://grants.nih.gov/grants/guide/notice-files/NOT-MH-02-001.html [accessed May 6, 2003]; *NIH Career Development Awards, Fiscal Year.* 2002. [Online]. Available: http://grants1.nih.gov/grants/award/training/careerdev02.htm [accessed May 6, 2003]; Henderson L, Lee B, Marino A. 2001. *Final Report On Three Focus Groups with Early Career Clinical Researchers about the K23 Award Program.* Washington, DC: AAMC.
[41] *APA/GlaxoSmithKline Young Faculty Award for Research Development in Biological Psychiatry.* [Online]. Available: http://www.psych.org/res_res/glaxo72001.cfm [accessed May 6, 2003].
[42] *Elaine Schlosser Lewis Pilot Research Award for Attention Disorder for a Junior Faculty of Child Psychiatrist Resident.* [Online]. Available: http://www.aacap.org/awards/esl.htm [accessed May 6, 2003].
[43] *2003 Bristol-Myers Squibb Fellowship.* [Online]. Available: http://www.acnp.org/graduate.php [accessed May 6, 2003].
[44] *Centers of Biomedical Research Excellence (COBRE).* [Online]. Available: http://grants1.nih.gov/grants/guide/rfa-files/RFA-RR-02-003.html [accessed May 6, 2003]; *Research Infrastructure – COBRE.* [Online]. Available: http://www.ncrr.nih.gov/resinfra/cobre.asp [accessed May 6, 2003]; *NCRR Fact Sheet.* [Online]. Available: http://www.ncrr.nih.gov/resinfra/ridea/ideafactsheet.pdf [accessed May 6, 2003].
[45] *Biomedical Research Infrastructure Network.* [Online]. Available: http://grants1.nih.gov/grants/guide/rfa-files/RFA-RR-01-005.html [accessed May 6, 2003]; *Research Infrastructure – BRIN.* [Online]. Available: http://www.ncrr.nih.gov/resinfra/brin.asp [accessed May 6, 2003]; *NCRR Fact Sheet.* [Online]. Available: http://www.ncrr.nih.gov/resinfra/riidea/ideafactsheet.pdf [accessed May 6, 2003].
[46] *Collaborative R01s for Clinical and Services Studies of Mental Disorders and AIDS.* [Online]. Available: http://grants1.nih.gov/grants/guide/pa-files/PA-01-123.html [accessed August 8, 2003]; *NIH Competing Research Project Applications.* [Online]. Available: http://grants2.nih.gov/grants/award/success/rpgicact9802.htm [accessed August 8, 2003].
[47] *NIMH Minority Research Infrastructure Support Program (R24).* [Online]. Available: http://grants1.nih.gov/grants/guide/pa-files/PAR-01-029.html [accessed May 30, 2003].

Appendix C

Brief Descriptions of Psychiatry Residency Training Programs*

* This is an illustrative list of programs. It is not intended as an exhaustive list, nor is it necessarily an endorsement of those programs listed.

Brief Descriptions of Psychiatry Residency Training Programs, Sorted by NIH 2002 Funding Rank for Each Department

Institution[a]	Research Track	Mentoring Program	No. of FTE Faculty M.D.s[b]	Elective Time[c]	No. of Residents[d]	Resident Compensation ($1000s)[e]		Other Notes	Research Rotation	FY2002 NIH Funding ($ millions, rank)	
						PGY1	PGY5			Psychiatry	Internal Medicine
WPIC (both)[1]	Y	Y	Adult: 111 Child: 25	PGY4: <12 mos PGY5: <12 mos	Adult: 61 Child: 13	37	42	22 residents are in the targeted research track; 7 T32 fellowships; the Junior Faculty Scholars Program has 8 slots to fund junior faculty 25% of time for 2 years to collect data for grant submissions – the program has yielded 11 career award submissions	Optional	77.5 (1)	43.6 (21)
Yale (both)[2]	Y	Y	Adult: 180 Child: 29	PGY2: 3 mos PGY4: 12 mos PGY5: 8 hrs/mo	Adult: 60 Child: 13	41.7	49.8	2 residents/year selected for Clinical Neuroscience Training Program that offers advanced research training; 184 patient-oriented research grants	Optional	39.1 (3)	52.7 (15)
Johns Hopkins (child)[3]	N	N	35	PGY6: ½ day/wk	12	43	46	—	Optional	33.3 (5)	137.0 (1)

Institution		Faculty	Research time			Description			
Washington University (both)[4]	Y	Adult: 67 Child: 6	PGY2: 50% for 4 mos PGY4: 8–10 mos PGY5: 20% for 8 mos	Adult: 38 Child: 6	37	42	45 R01 grants, 14 K awards, and 6 training grants; 27 research fellows; offers a master degree in psychiatric epidemiology	Optional	33.3 (6)	62.0 (11)
Duke (both)[5]	Y	Adult: 171 Child: 12	PGY3: 4–12 hrs/wk PGY4: 4–20 hrs/wk	Adult: 43 Child: 8	37	44	—	Negotiable in adult; optional in child	32.9 (7)	80.0 (6)
UCSD (both)[6]	Y	Adult: 50 Child: 9	PGY4: 12 mos PGY5: 0	Adult: 36 Child: 8	37	47	Research requirement for residents; 2–3 residents enter research track (began in 1998) – research time of 20% in PGY3 and 75% in PGY4; 3 NIMH-funded clinical research centers	Optional	26.2 (8)	80.0 (5)
Stanford (both)[7]	Y	Adult: 45 Child: 8	PGY4: 9 mos	Adult: 45	41	51	Research track available to 2 residents-research time of 25% in PGY3 and 80% in PGY4	Optional for adult	21.3 (9)	44.6 (20)
Columbia (both)[8]	Y	Adult: 120 Child: 59	PGY4: 65% PGY5: 15% for 6 mos	Adult: 47 Child: 13	43	73	9 separate postresidency research training programs	Optional	20.0 (10)	46.1 (17)

Continued

Brief Descriptions of Psychiatry Residency Training Programs, Sorted by NIH 2002 Funding Rank for Each Department

Institution[a]	Research Track	Mentoring Program	No. of FTE Faculty M.D.s[b]	Elective Time[c]	No. of Residents[d]	Resident Compensation ($1000s)[e]		Other Notes	Research Rotation	FY2002 NIH Funding ($ millions, rank)	
						PGY1	PGY5			Psychiatry	Internal Medicine
UCLA–Harbor (both)[9]	N	N[f]	25	PGY4: 40%	28	36	50	NIMH Minority Mental Health Research Unit	Optional	19.1 (11)	71.7 (8)
UCLA–Neuropsychiatric Institute (child)[10]	N	Y	20	PGY5: 5 hrs/wk	12	37	47	1–2 yr NIMH-funded research fellowship for M.D.'s or Ph.D.'s	Negotiable	19.1 (11)	71.7 (8)
University of Texas at Southwestern (both)*[11]	Y	Y	Adult: 80 Child: 8	PGY4: 7 mos PGY5: 15%	Adult: 61 Child: 10	35	42	7 residents on the research track; those completing the research track are recruited as junior faculty	Optional for adult	18.6 (13)	46.5 (16)
University of Colorado (child)[12]	Y	Y	20	PGY4: 6 hrs/wk PGY5: 15 hrs/wk	9	38	47	6 research institutes; T32 training grant	Optional	13.8 (17)	57.4 (14)

Institution										
Emory (both)*[13]	N	Y	Adult: 60 Child: 8–10	PGY4: 8 mos PGY5: <2 mos	Adult: 50 Child: 8	39	45	Pending R25 to fund formal research track; offers a masters degree in clinical research through the School of Public Health	Optional	13.7 (18)	26.8 (34)
NYU (child)[14]	Y	Y	21	PGY5: 1 day/wk for 3 mos	12	45	53	Residents exposed to research in PGY2; NIMH-funded fellowship available	Optional	9.6 (26)	20.3 (43)
University of Michigan (adult)[15]	Y	Y	50	4-yr track: 8–9 mos 5-yr track: 2–3 mos	48	37	45	50% of academic track residents have M.D./Ph.D.; R25 mechanism provides 18 months of research training as part of 5-year residency	Optional	9.6 (27)	66.3 (10)
Wayne State (both)[16]	Y[g] N[h]	N[i]	Adult: 31 Child: 8	PGY3: ½ day/wk for 12 mos PGY4: 5 mos PGY5: 2 mos	Adult: 24 Child: 6	39	44	Adult psychiatry residents are required to produce a scholarly paper and present at grand rounds; masters of science in psychiatry	Optional	7.6 (28)	13.0 (55)
University of Maryland (both)[17]	Y	Y	Adult: 49 Child: 3	PGY4: 12 mos PGY5: 0	Adult: 74 Child: 10	37	43	NIMH-funded research track extends residency to 5 years	Optional	7.3 (31)	32.5 (30)
University of Minnesota (both)*[18]	Y	Y	Adult: 29 Child: 4	PGY4: 12 mos PGY5: 3 mos	Adult: 33 Child: 6	38	44	—	Optional	6.4 (33)	28.2 (33)

Continued

Brief Descriptions of Psychiatry Residency Training Programs, Sorted by NIH 2002 Funding Rank for Each Department

Institution[a]	Research Track	Mentoring Program	No. of FTE Faculty M.D.s[b]	Elective Time[c]	No. of Residents[d]	Resident Compensation ($1000s)[e]		Other Notes	Research Rotation	FY2002 NIH Funding ($ millions, rank)	
						PGY1	PGY5			Psychiatry	Internal Medicine
University of Vermont (adult)[19]	Y	Y	21	PGY4: 8 mos	16	39	N/A	Behavioral Genetics Research Division; Center For Children, Youth, and Families; Clinical Neuroscience Research Unit; Human Behavioral Psychopharmacology Unit; 14 R01 grants; department ranked 2nd in funding at university; 11 research fellows	Optional	6.0 (34)	14.0 (51)
Indiana University (both)*[20]	N	N	Adult: 28 Child: 8	PGY2–PGY4: <12 mos PGY5: N/A	Adult: 24 Child: 8	38	40	Research-minded residents recruited as junior faculty; pending NIH application for a research track	Negotiable in adult; optional for child	5.2 (37)	41.3 (22)
Virginia Commonwealth University	N	Y	Adult: 35 Child: 8	PGY4: 10–20 hrs/wk for 8 mos; PGY4 (Child): Y	Adult: 36 Child: 6	36	39	Required research activity	Optional for adult	4.9 (39)	14.3 (50)

237

Institution											
Dartmouth (both)[22]	N	Y	Adult: 44 Child: 6	PGY4: 6 mos PGY5: 1.5 mos	Adult: 27 Child: 6^i	41	47	—	Optional	4.8 (40)	12.7 (56)
University of Connecticut (both)[23]	N	Y	Adult: 31 Child: 5	PGY4 (Adult): 40% PGY4 (Child): 2 mos	Adult: 28 Child: 6	40	44	$10 million research budget; research requirement; provides intense one-on-one didactic research training to young investigators	Required	4.6 (41)	9.7 (64)
University of Arkansas (both)*[24]	Y	Y	Adult: 54 Child: 10	PGY4: 12 mos PGY5: 23%	Adult: 24 Child: 4	34	39	—	Optional	4.2 (42)	7.5 (69)
Ohio State University (both)[25]	N	N	Adult: 16 Child: 3.5	PGY2: 1 mos PGY4: 5 mos PGY5: 0	Adult: 20 Child: 2	38	44	$15 million neuropsychiatric facility opened in 1994	Optional for adult	3.6 (45)	24.3 (37)
UMDNJ–Newark (both)[26]	N	N	Adult: <43 Child: 6	PGY4: <8 mos PGY5: <6 mos	Adult: 30 Child: 4	41	51	Planning to implement one-on-one mentorship; hosts an annual research day	Optional for adult; 26 wks required rotation for child	3.3 (47)	6.0 (74)
Brown (both)*[27]	Y	Y	Adult: 30 Child: 14	PGY4: 6–8 mos PGY5: 60% for 4 mos	Adult: 40 Child: 10	39	46	1–2 residents/yr on the research track; tracks residents after graduating; has two T32 programs; hosts annual research day	Optional in adult; 1 wk required in child	2.7 (51)	1.1 (100)

Continued

Brief Descriptions of Psychiatry Residency Training Programs, Sorted by NIH 2002 Funding Rank for Each Department

Institution[a]	Research Track	Mentoring Program	No. of FTE Faculty M.D.s[b]	Elective Time[c]	No. of Residents[d]	Resident Compensation ($1000s)[e]		Other Notes	Research Rotation	FY2002 NIH Funding ($ millions, rank)	
						PGY1	PGY5			Psychiatry	Internal Medicine
Howard (adult)[28]	N	Y	17	PGY4: 5–9 mos	15	35	40	Faculty have received $6 million for mood and anxiety studies from NIH; site for NIMH-funded Systematic Treatment Enhancement Program for Bipolar Disorder	Optional	1.2 (65)	3.6 (80)
Thomas Jefferson University (adult)[29]	Y	N	17	PGY4: 6 mos	28	38	—	Research Scholars Program for physician-scientists, Training Program in Human Investigation	Optional	0.99 (71)	21.3 (41)
Wake Forest (both)[30]	N	N	Adult: 12 Child: 3	PGY4: 6 mos PGY5: N/A	Adult: 23 Child: 3	37	39	1 K23 grant, 2 career awards, 1 APA award, 5 pharmaceutical grants, 8 additional grants through NIMH, 1 NICHD grant; NIMH-funded Research Infrastructure Support Program	Optional for adult	0.92 (72)	15.9 (46)

238

Program											
Medical College of Georgia (child)[31]	N	Y	6	0	4	36	40	Residents must complete a research paper	Negotiable	0.72 (76)	2.9 (84)
SUNY–Buffalo (child)[32]	N	Y	9	<6 mos	6	34	38	Research project required; research involvement for 2 hrs/wk in PGY4 and 6 weeks full-time in PGY5	Negotiable	0.46 (79)	4.4 (79)
Texas A&M (both)[33]	N	N	Adult: 27 Child: 4	PGY4: 8 mos PGY5: 30% for 6 mos	Adult: 16 Child: 4	36	41	Adult program began in 1993; child program began in 1998	Optional	0.35 (80)	0.17 (110)
Elmhurst Hospital Center (adult)[34]	N	Y	34	PGY4: 6–8 mos	28	~40s	—	Institute for Cultural and Epidemiological Psychiatry	Optional	N/A	N/A
Maine Medical Center (both)[35]	N	N	Adult: 15 Child: 5	PGY4: 4 mos PGY5: 0	Adult: 16 Child: 4	40	48	Required scholarly project	Optional for adult	N/A	N/A
Mayo Clinic (both)[36]	Y	Y	Adult: 39 Child: 8	PGY4: 6 mos PGY5: <4 mos	Adult: 31 Child: 6	39	45	Offers the Clinician-Investigator Training program—masters degree, formal training in basic and clinical research	Optional	N/A	N/A

Continued

Brief Descriptions of Psychiatry Residency Training Programs, Sorted by NIH 2002 Funding Rank for Each Department

Institution[a]	Research Track	Mentoring Program	No. of FTE Faculty M.D.s[b]	Elective Time[c]	No. of Residents[d]	Resident Compensation ($1000s)[e]		Other Notes	Research Rotation	FY2002 NIH Funding ($ millions, rank)	
						PGY1	PGY5			Psychiatry	Internal Medicine
Med College Ohio (child)[37]	N	N	3	2	4	39	45	Research/review paper required	Optional	N/A	1.1 (101)
Michigan State University–Kalamazoo Center (adult)[38]	N	Y	11	PGY4: 6 mos	16	38	42	Residency program began in 1997; residents must be involved in a research project by either designing their own small study or joining and participating in larger faculty projects	Optional	N/A	N/A
North Dakota (adult)[39]	Y	Y	4	PGY4: <12 mos	16	39	—	$22 million endowment for Neuropsychiatry Research Institute	Optional	N/A	N/A
St. Luke's Hospital (both)[40]	Y	N	Adult: 79	PGY4: 6 mos PGY5: 1 day/wk for 4 mos	Adult: 32	46	—	Two residents chosen for research track beginning in PGY3; research electives may be carried out in the department, with a member of Columbia University or at an affiliated institution	Optional for adult	N/A	N/A

Institution								
Southern Illinois University (adult)[41]	N	N	15	PGY4: 9 mos	12 (10 Internal medicine/ psychiatry)	40	46	Residents interested in research collaborate with research director	Optional	N/A	0.09 (111)
University of Louisville (both)[42]	N	N	Adult: 36 Child: 6	PGY4: 3 mos PGY5: <4 mos	Adult: 36 Child: 4	37	45	About 25% of faculty actively engaged in research; Mood Disorders Research Program; Clinical Psychopharmacology Research Program	Optional	N/A	7.0 (70)
University of Nebraska (both)*[43]	N	N	Adult: 29 Child: 7	PGY4: <4 mos	Adult: 24 Child: 4	39	45	—	Optional for adult; 2 wks required rotation for child	N/A	2.4 (91)

NOTES: APA = American Psychiatric Association; FTE = full-time equivalent; M.D. = medical doctor/doctor of medicine; NICHD = National Institute of Child Health and Human Development; NIH = National Institutes of Health; NIMH = National Institute of Mental Health; WPIC = Western Psychiatric Institute and Clinic; NYU = New York University; PGY = postgraduate year; SUNY = State University of New York; UCLA = University of California, Los Angeles; UCSD = University of California, San Diego; UMDNJ = University of Medicine & Dentistry of New Jersey; * = Departments whose chairs were interviewed

[a] "Both" refers to adult (general) psychiatry and child and adolescent psychiatry residency programs. In cases where both residencies are discussed, the table lists separately: the number of full-time equivalent M.D. faculty, amount of elective time, number of residents, level of compensation, and research rotation requirements.

[b] Information obtained from the *American Medical Association's (AMA) Fellowship and Residency Electronic Interactive Database (FREIDA)*. [Online]. Available: http://www.ama-assn.org/vapp/freida/srch/1,2667,Y,00.html [accessed January 17, 2003], unless specifically provided by department staff or chairs who were interviewed.

[c] Information obtained primarily from the American Psychiatric Association's *Directory of Psychiatry Residency Training Programs (Seventh Edition)*. 1997. Washington, DC and from the psychiatry department's website if information was unavailable in that source. PGY2, PGY3, and PGY4 refer to the adult (general) psychiatry program, and PGY5 and PGY6 refers to the child and adolescent psychiatry program, unless otherwise indicated. The symbol "Y" for "yes" is given if elective time is available, but it is not clear how much time is allocated, and "N/A" denotes "not available" if the information was not provided or could not be found.

[d] Information obtained from FREIDA (see note b).

[e] As with note d.

NOTES continued for Brief Descriptions of Psychiatry Residency Training Programs

f Informal.
g For adult.
h For child/adolescent.
i The University of Vermont shares a child and adolescent residency with Dartmouth. There are two child and adolescent psychiatry residents at Dartmouth, which serves as the primary site.
j The University of Connecticut shares a child and adolescent residency with the Institute of Living.

SOURCES:

[1] Personal communication, P. Pilkonis, WPIC, March 10, 2003; personal communication, N. Ryan, WPIC, April 16, 2003, April 17, 2003; Pilkonis PA. 2001 (November 7). *Pittsburgh Model: Early Faculty Development (R25 Model)*. National Institute of Mental Health and the American Psychiatric Association Workshop on Research Training for Psychiatrists. Bethesda, MD; Swartz HA, Cho RY. 2002 (Fall). *Building Bridges: The Pittsburgh Model of Research Career Development, Psychiatric Research Report; Western Psychiatric Institute and Clinic*. [Online]. Available: http://www.wpic.pitt.edu/ [accessed May 6, 2003].

[2] Personal communication, S. Bunney, Yale University, June 17, 2003; personal communication, D. Stubbe, Yale University, June 19, 2003; *Yale University Department of Psychiatry*. [Online]. Available: http://info.med.yale.edu/psych/welcome.html [accessed May 6, 2003].

[3] Personal communication, E. Frosch, Johns Hopkins University, February 20, 2003, March 10, 2003; *Johns Hopkins University Department of Psychiatry and Behavioral Sciences*. [Online]. Available: http://www.hopkinsmedicine.org/jhhpsychiatry/master1.htm [accessed May 6, 2003].

[4] Hudziak, J. 2002 (June 20). *The Implications of Size, Culture, RRC, and Funding on Psychiatric Research Training in Residency: University of Washington and the University of Vermont*. Presentation at the Institute of Medicine Committee on Incorporating Research into Psychiatry Residency Training. Washington, DC; *Washington University St. Louis Department of Psychiatry*. [Online]. Available: www.psychiatry.wustl.edu [accessed May 6, 2003].

[5] Personal communication, G. Thrall, Duke University, April 2, 2003; March JS. 2002 (June 19). *Research Training in Child Psychiatry*. Presentation at the Institute of Medicine Workshop for the Committee on Incorporating Research into Psychiatry Residency Training. Washington, DC; *Duke University Department of Psychiatry*. [Online]. Available: http://www.psychres.duke.edu [accessed May 6, 2003].

[6] Personal communication, S. Zisook, UCSD, February 11, 2003, April 3, 2003; *UCSD Residency Training Program*. [Online]. Available: http://residenttraining.ucsd.edu/ [accessed May 6, 2003].

[7] Personal communication, F. Sloss, Stanford University, March 6, 2003; Meyer RE, McLaughlin CJ. 1998. *Between Mind, Brain, and Managed Care*. Washington, DC: APA; *Stanford University Department of Psychiatry*. [Online]. Available: http://psychiatry.stanford.edu/ [accessed May 6, 2003].

[8] Shaffer D. 2002 (June 19). *Child Psychiatry's Perspective: Part I*. Presentation at the Institute of Medicine Workshop of the Committee on Incorporating Research into Psychiatry Residency Training. Washington, DC; personal communication, R. Rieder, Columbia University, April 10, 2003, April 11, 2003; personal communication, J. Dierkens, Columbia University, April 9, 2003; *Columbia University Department of Psychiatry*. [Online]. Available: http://cpmcnet.columbia.edu/dept/pi/psychres/psychfront-gd.html [accessed May 6, 2003].

NOTES continued for Brief Descriptions of Psychiatry Residency Training Programs

[9] Personal communication, I. Lesser, UCLA-Harbor, February 25, 2003, April 2, 2003; *Harbor-UCLA Medical Center Department of Psychiatry.* [Online]. Available: http://www.harboruclapsych.com/home.htm [accessed May 6, 2003].

[10] Personal communication, B. Zima, UCLA-NPI, February 10, 2003; personal communication, K. Nelson, UCLA-NPI, March 27, 2003; *UCLA Department of Psychiatry.* [Online]. Available: http://www.psychiatry.ucla.edu/index.html [accessed May 6, 2003].

[11] Personal communication, E. Nestler, University of Texas at Southwestern, November 7, 2002, February 11, 2003, May 28, 2003; *The University of Texas at Southwestern Medical Center at Dallas Department of Psychiatry.* [Online]. Available: http://www3.utsouthwestern.edu/psychiatry [accessed May 6, 2003].

[12] Personal communication, D. Carter, University of Colorado, February 11, 2003; personal communication, R. Harmon, University of Colorado, February 10, 2003; Meyer RE, McLaughlin CJ. 1998. *Between Mind, Brain, and Managed Care.* Washington, DC: APA; *University of Colorado Department of Psychiatry.* [Online]. Available: http://www.uchsc.edu/sm/psych/dept/index.htm [accessed May 6, 2003].

[13] Personal communication, C. Nemeroff, Emory University, November 21, 2002; personal communication, M. Crowder, Emory University, March 28, 2003; personal communication, P. Haugaard, Emory University, March 28, 2003; *Emory University Department of Psychiatry and Behavioral Sciences.* [Online]. Available: http://www.psychiatry.emory.edu/ [accessed May 6, 2003].

[14] Personal communication, C. Alonso, New York University, March 27, 2003; *New York University Department of Psychiatry.* [Online]. Available: http://www.med.nyu.edu/Psych/ [accessed May 6, 2003].

[15] Personal communication, M. Jibson, University of Michigan, February 11, 2003; Meador-Woodruff JH. 2001 (November 7). *Residency Research Track Program (R25 Model).* National Institute of Mental Health and the American Psychiatric Association Workshop on Research Training for Psychiatrists. Bethesda, MD; *University of Michigan Department of Psychiatry.* [Online]. Available: http://www.med.umich.edu/psych/ [accessed May 6, 2003].

[16] Personal communication, B. Brooks, Wayne State University, February 10, 2003; *Wayne State University Department of Psychiatry.* [Online]. Available: http://www.med.wayne.edu/psychiatry/ [accessed May 6, 2003].

[17] Personal communication, M. P. Luber, University of Maryland, April 7, 2003; *Sheppard Pratt Health System.* [Online]. Available: http://www.sheppardpratt.org [accessed May 6, 2003]; *University of Maryland/Sheppard Pratt Psychiatry Residency Program.* [Online]. Available: http://www.umm.edu/psychiatry/ [accessed May 6, 2003].

[18] Personal communication, C. Schulz, November 22, 2002; personal communication, T. Mackenzie, University of Minnesota, November 22, 2002; *University of Minnesota Department of Psychiatry.* [Online]. Available: http://www.med.umn.edu/psychiatry/ [accessed May 6, 2003].

[19] Hudziak, J. 2002 (June 20). *The Implications of Size, Culture, RRC, and Funding on Psychiatric Research Training in Residency: University of Washington and the University of Vermont.* Presentation at the Institute of Medicine Committee on Incorporating Research into Psychiatry Residency Training. Washington, DC; personal communication, J. Hudziak, University of Vermont, March 30, 2003; *University of Vermont* [Online]. Available: http://www.vtmednet.org/psychiatry/ [accessed May 6, 2003].

[20] Personal communication, C. McDougle, Indiana University, November 4, 2002, February 10, 2003; *Indiana University Department of Psychiatry.* [Online]. Available: http://www.iupui.edu/~psycdept [accessed May 6, 2003].

NOTES *continued for* Brief Descriptions of Psychiatry Residency Training Programs

[21] Personal communication, J. Silverman, Virginia Commonwealth University, November 5, 2002, February 19, 2003; *Virginia Commonwealth University Department of Psychiatry.* [Online]. Available: http://views.vcu.edu/psych/ [accessed May 6, 2003].

[22] Personal communication, R. Racusin, Dartmouth University, February 11, 2003, personal communication, J. Hudziak, University of Vermont, March 30, 2003; Meyer RE, McLaughlin CJ. 1998. *Between Mind, Brain, and Managed Care.* Washington, DC: APA; *Dartmouth-Hitchcock Medical Center.* [Online]. Available: http://www.hitchcock.org/ [accessed May 6, 2003].

[23] Personal communication, L. Huey, University of Connecticut, October 3, 2002, February 14, 2003, July 30, 2003; *University of Connecticut Department of Psychiatry.* [Online]. Available: http://psychiatry.uchc.edu/index.php [accessed May 6, 2003].

[24] Personal communication, G. R. Smith, University of Arkansas, December 5, 2002, March 30, 2003; *Division of Child and Adolescent Psychiatry Residency Program Manual 2002-2003* [Online]. Available: http://www.childpsych.uams.edu/Residency%20Manual/RM%2002-03.pdf [accessed May 6, 2003]; *UAMS Department of Psychiatry.* [Online]. Available: http://www.uams.edu/psych/ [accessed May 6, 2003].

[25] Personal communication, H. Nasrallah, Veterans Administration Medical Center, July 29, 2003; *Ohio State University Department of Psychiatry.* [Online]. Available: http://medicine.osu.edu/psychiatry/ [accessed May 6, 2003].

[26] Personal communication, C. Kellner, UMDNJ–New Jersey Medical School at Newark, November 12, 2002; *UMDNJ Psychiatry Residency Training Program.* [Online]. Available: http://njms.umdnj.edu/psychiatry/residency/index.htm [accessed May 6, 2003].

[27] Personal communication, M. Keller, Brown University, November 20, 2002; personal communication, T. Mueller, Brown University, November 20, 2002, March 28, 2003; personal communication, H. Leonard, Brown University, November 20, 2002; *Brown University Department of Psychiatry & Human Behavior.* [Online]. Available: http://www.neuropsychiatry.com/DPHB/ [accessed May 6, 2003].

[28] Lawson, W. 2002 (June 20). *Howard University.* Presentation at the Institute of Medicine Committee on Incorporating Research into Psychiatry Residency Training. Washington, DC; personal communication, J. Hutchinson, Howard University, May 5, 2003; *Howard University Department of Psychiatry.* [Online]. Available: http://www.huhosp.org/psychiatry/index.htm [accessed May 6, 2003].

[29] Personal communication, E. Silberman, Thomas Jefferson University, February 10, 2003; *Thomas Jefferson University Department of Psychiatry and Human Behavior.* [Online]. Available: http://www.tju.edu/psych/home/index.cfm [accessed May 6, 2003].

[30] Personal communication, S. Kramer, Wake Forest University, February 12, 2003; *Wake Forest University Department of Psychiatry.* [Online]. Available: http://www.wfubmc.edu/psychiatry/ [accessed May 6, 2003].

[31] *Medical College of Georgia General Psychiatry Residency Program.* [Online]. Available: http://www.mcg.edu/Resident/psychiatry/Index.htm [accessed May 6, 2003].

[32] Personal communication, D. L. Kaye, SUNY-University of Buffalo, April 3, 2003; *SUNY-University of Buffalo Department of Psychiatry.* [Online]. Available: http://www.smbs.buffalo.edu/psychiatry/main/index.html [accessed May 6, 2003].

[33] Personal communication, J. Ripperger-Suhler, Texas A&M University Scott & White Clinic, April 22, 2003; *Texas A&M University Graduate Medical Education.* [Online]. Available: http://www.sw.org/gme/welcome.htm [accessed May 6, 2003].

[34] Personal communication, A. Hoffman, Elmhurst Hospital, February 10, 2003; *Elmhurst Hospital.* [Online]. Available:

NOTES continued for Brief Descriptions of Psychiatry Residency Training Programs

[35]Personal communication, G. McNeil, Maine Medical Center, April 4, 2003; *Maine Medical Center General Psychiatry Residency Training*. [Online]. Available: http://www.mmc.org/residencies/psychiatry/default.htm [accessed May 6, 2003].

[36]Personal communication, G. Rink, Mayo Clinic, March 27, 2003; *Mayo Clinic*. [Online]. Available: http://mayoclinic.org [accessed May 6, 2003].

[37]Personal communication, W. J. Kim, Medical College of Ohio, February 10, 2003; *Medical College of Ohio Department of Psychiatry*. [Online]. Available: http://www.mco.edu/depts/psych/ [accessed May 6, 2003]

[38]Personal communication, M. Liepman, Michigan State University-Kalamazoo Center, February 11, 2003; *Michigan State University-Kalamazoo Center Psychiatry Residency Program*. [Online]. Available: http://www.kcms.msu.edu/programs/psychiatry/index.html [accessed May 6, 2003].

[39]Personal communication, D. Abbott, University of North Dakota, April 10, 2003; *UND Psychiatry Residency Training Program*. [Online]. Available: http://www.med.und.nodak.edu/residency/residency/psychiatry.html [accessed May 6, 2003].

[40]*St. Luke's–Roosevelt Department of Psychiatry*. [Online]. Available: www.wehealny.org/psych/residency.html [accessed May 6, 2003].

[41]Personal communication, S. Soltys, Southern Illinois University, February 14, 2003; *SIU Department of Psychiatry*. [Online]. Available: http://www.siumed.edu/medpsy/ [accessed May 6, 2003].

[42]Personal communication, K. Vincent, University of Louisville, February 26, 2003; Meyer RE, McLaughlin CJ. 1998. *Between Mind, Brain, and Managed Care*. Washington, DC: APA; *University of Louisville Department of Psychiatry and Behavioral Sciences*. [Online]. Available: http://www.louisville.edu/medschool/psychiatry/ [accessed May 6, 2003].

[43]Personal communication, D. Folks, University of Nebraska, November 18, 2002, April 16, 2003; *University of Nebraska Department of Psychiatry*. [Online]. Available: http://www.unmc.edu/psychiatry/ [accessed May 6, 2003].

Appendix D

Committee and Staff Biographies

COMMITTEE

THOMAS BOAT, M.D. *(Chair)*, is director of the Children's Hospital Research Foundation and Professor and chair in the department of pediatrics within the University of Cincinnati. He has served on the certification committee of the American Board of Medical Specialties (1998–2000), as chair for a task force on the future of pediatric education (1996–1999), and as president for the American Pediatric Society (1999–2000). Dr. Boat is a pediatric pulmonologist by training and has a research background in the molecular pathophysiology of lung diseases, especially cystic fibrosis. His current interests and involvements are in the areas of (1) redesign of graduate medical education; (2) improvements in the delivery of child health care, including the creation of hospital–community partnerships; and (3) management of academic health centers, with emphasis on the application of business approaches to maximize resource utilization for program development and maintenance.

BARBARA ATKINSON, M.D., is executive dean and vice chancellor for clinical affairs at the University of Kansas School of Medicine. She was previously professor, chair, and residency program director in the Department of Pathology and Laboratory Medicine at the University of Kansas in Kansas City, and prior to that had served as Annenberg Dean of MCP Hahnemann School of Medicine (1996–1999). She is a trustee (1991–present) and past president (1998) of the American Board of Pathology. Dr. Atkinson was previously a member of the Pathology Residency Review Committee (1992–1996) of the Accreditation Council for Graduate Medical Education. Her research has been in the identification and characterization of tumor antigens in cells and tissues and in the development of techniques to recognize tumors and tumor types. Dr. Atkinson has edited several books in cytopathology and gynecologic pathology, including one of the classic books in the discipline, the *Atlas of Cytopathology*, published in 1992, and the *Atlas of Difficult Diagnosis in Cytopathology*, published in 1998 by Saunders. She recently served on an Association of American Medical Colleges Committee on Increasing Women's Leadership in Academic Medicine.

BENJAMIN S. BUNNEY, M.D., is Charles B. G. Murphy Professor and chair of the department of psychiatry, professor of pharmacology, and professor of neurobiology at the Yale Medical School. Dr. Bunney is one of the world's leading experts on the brain's dopamine systems, whose malfunctioning has been implicated in the pathogenesis of schizophrenia and neurological movement disorders, such as Parkinson's disease. He is a past president of the American College of Neuropsychopharmacology and the recipient of its highest research award, the Daniel H. Efron Award. He was also the first recipient of the Lieber Prize for outstanding achievement in research on mental illness from the National Alliance for Research on Schizophrenia and Depression. Dr. Bunney serves on numerous editorial boards and pharmaceutical company scientific advisory boards, and is a member of the Institute of Medicine.

GABRIELLE A. CARLSON, M.D., has been professor of psychiatry and pediatrics and director of the division of child and adolescent psychiatry at the State University of New York at Stony Brook since 1985. Dr. Carlson specializes in childhood psychopathology and psychopharmacology in general, and in the subjects of childhood and adolescent depression and bipolar disorder more specifically. She has written more than 150 papers and chapters on those subjects and has coauthored two books: *Affective Disorders in Childhood Adolescence* (Spectrum Publications) and *Psychiatric Disorders in Children and Adolescents* (W. B. Saunders). Her research interests include the phenomenology and long-term follow-up of young people with bipolar disorder, and the relationship of behavior disorders and mood disorders. Her most recent grants have focused on those questions. Dr. Carlson has been named among the Best Doctors in America and *Good Housekeeping's* Best Mental Health Experts. She has served on several editorial boards (*Journal of the American Academy of Child and Adolescent Psychiatry, American Journal of Psychiatry, Journal of*

Affective Disorders, Journal of Child and Adolescent Psychopharmacology) and numerous professional committees.

JAMES J. HUDZIAK, M.D., is an associate professor of psychiatry and medicine and director of child psychiatry in the department of psychiatry at the University of Vermont. He also serves as director of the division of behavioral genetics and research director of pediatric psychopharmacology. In addition, he has an adjunct appointment as associate professor of psychiatry at Dartmouth Medical School. His research efforts have involved the study of genetic factors influencing social behaviors, attention, and aggression. His funded research has included phenotypic, endophenotypic, and molecular genetic and pharmacologic studies of child psychopathology. Dr. Hudziak has published numerous peer-reviewed articles, reviews articles for a number of journals, and reviews grants for the National Institute of Mental Health as well as the Dutch National and Scottish National Review Boards. He also has been heavily involved in medical student and residency education in psychiatry and genetics. He has served on two Josiah Macy Foundation studies on the importance of genetics and on psychiatry education in medicine. He is a member of a number of professional organizations, such as the American Psychiatric Association, the American Academy of Child and Adolescent Psychiatry, the Behavioral Genetics Association, the International Society of Psychiatric Genetics, and the Society of Professors in Child and Adolescent Psychiatry.

DEAN KILPATRICK, Ph.D., is a professor of psychiatry and behavioral sciences at the Medical University of South Carolina in Charleston. He received a Ph.D. in clinical psychology from the University of Georgia in 1970 and has been a faculty member at the Medical University since receiving his degree. Throughout his career, Dr. Kilpatrick has been an active researcher and has received numerous peer-reviewed extramural research grants from a host of federal agencies. For the past 14 years, he has been principal investigator on a National Institute of Mental Health–funded research-training grant that provides scientist-practitioner research training to three predoctoral and three postdoctoral students each year. He is also editor of the *Journal of Traumatic Stress*, a multidisciplinary international journal. For the past 20 years, Dr. Kilpatrick has served as director or codirector of the Charleston Consortium Clinical Psychology Internship Program. Throughout his career, he has been involved in a variety of educational activities with medical students and psychiatry residents. Dr. Kilpatrick also has experience in the area of public policy. He has provided invited testimony about public policy issues to committees of the United States House and Senate, state legislatures, and federal courts. He has also served on various committees tasked with making research-based policy recommendations to federal agencies.

WILLIAM LAWSON, M.D., is currently professor and chairman of the department of psychiatry at Howard University School of Medicine. He is also chair of the section of psychiatry and behavioral sciences of the National Medical Association. He is past president of the Black Psychiatrists of America. Dr. Lawson has produced more than 85 publications involving severe mental illness and its relationship to psychopharmacology, substance abuse, and racial and ethnic issues. He has a long-standing concern with ethnic disparities in mental health treatment and has been an outspoken advocate for access to services among the severely mentally ill. He currently is a member of the Scientific Advisory Committee, National Depression and Manic Depressive Society, and on the boards of the DC Mental Health Association and DC Alliance for the Mentally Ill. He is currently directing a $6.5 million contract with the National Institute of Mental Health intramural program to conduct research on mood and anxiety disorders among African Americans and other ethnic minorities.

VIRGINIA MAN-YEE LEE, Ph.D., is professor of pathology and laboratory medicine and director of the Center for Neurodegenerative Disease Research at the University of Pennsylvania School of Medicine, and is the first recipient of the John H. Ware III Chair for Alzheimer's Disease Research. Dr. Lee's research focuses on the pathogenesis of Alzheimer's disease, Parkinson's disease, frontotemporal dementia, and related neurodegenerative disorders of aging. Since 1970, she has authored over 400 papers, including more than 200 papers on Alzheimer's disease, pulmonary disease, and other age-related neurodegenerative disorders. She was elected a councilor in the Society for Neuroscience (2001) and continues to serve on a number of grant review committees, including NIH study sections and foundation review committees, such as that of the Alzheimer's Association.

JEROME POSNER, M.D., is currently George C. Cotzias Chair of Neuro-Oncology at the Memorial Sloan-Kettering Cancer Center and an American Cancer Society research professor. He was chair of the department of neurology at Sloan-Kettering from 1975 to 1997. His current research is on the biology of paraneoplastic syndromes—

disorders of an organ or tissue caused by cancer, but not a direct effect of the tumor or a metastasis to the involved organ.

DAVID REISS, M.D., is Vivian Gill Distinguished Professor and director of the division of research in the department of psychiatry and behavioral sciences at The George Washington University. He has been at The George Washington University since 1974. Between 1966 and 1974, he served in various positions in the adult psychiatry branch at the National Institute of Mental Health including section chief and acting branch chief. Dr. Reiss' current research focuses on mechanisms of gene–environment interplay in children, adolescents, and adults. He directs a National Institute of Mental Health–supported training grant that includes programs for attracting psychiatric residents into research and has mentored numerous K awards for early career research psychiatrists. Dr. Reiss has received many research awards, including a National Institute of Mental Health merit award; this year he will receive the Adolf Meyer Award from the American Psychiatric Association. He is a member of the Institute of Medicine's Board of Neurosciences and Behavioral Health.

MICHELLE RIBA, M.D, M.S., is clinical professor and associate chair for education and academic affairs in the department of psychiatry, University of Michigan Health System, and director of the psycho-oncology program at the University of Michigan Comprehensive Cancer Center. Dr. Riba has served as vice president, secretary, and trustee at large for the American Psychiatric Association and in May 2003 became president-elect. She is past president of the American Association of Directors of Psychiatric Residency Training and the Association for Academic Psychiatry. Dr. Riba is a fellow in the Class of 2002–2003 Hedwig van Ameringen Executive Leadership in Academic Medicine Program for Women. She has coedited 13 editions of *The American Psychiatric Press Review of Psychiatry* series. She has also coedited *Psychopharmacology and Psychotherapy: A Collaborative Approach; Primary Care Psychiatry; and The Doctor-Patient Relationship in Pharmacotherapy: Improving Treatment Effectiveness.* Dr. Riba is the author or coauthor of more than 100 scientific articles, chapters, and scientific abstracts. Her research interests are in psycho-oncology and the integration of psychotherapy and pharmacotherapy.

RICHARD SCHEFFLER, Ph.D., is distinguished professor of health economics and public policy at the University of California, Berkeley, and holds the chair in healthcare markets and consumer welfare endowed by the Office of the Attorney General for the State of California. He is director of the Petris Center. At Berkeley, he serves as codirector of the Scholars in Health Policy Research Program, funded by The Robert Wood Johnson Foundation. He is founding codirector of the National Institute of Mental Health pre- and postdoctoral training programs. He also codirects the National Institutes of Health–Fogarty Mental Health and Policy Research Training for Czech Post Doctoral Scholars program; the Agency for Healthcare Research and Quality pre- and postdoctoral training program; and the Edmund S. Muskie Fellowship Program. He served as president and program chair of the International Health Economics Association (iHEA) Fourth World Congress in San Francisco, June 2003. His research is on health care markets, health insurance, the health workforce, mental health economics, and international health system reforms in Western and Eastern Europe. He is the recipient of a senior scientist award from National Institute of Mental Health for studying mental health. Professor Scheffler has been a Fulbright Scholar, a Rockefeller Scholar, and a Scholar in Residence at the Institute of Medicine–National Academy of Sciences. He has published more than 125 papers and edited and written six books. His forthcoming book (University of California Press) is on the future of the health workforce.

JOEL YAGER, M.D., is professor of psychiatry and vice chair for education at the University of New Mexico School of Medicine and is professor of psychiatry emeritus at the University of California at Los Angeles. His research and scholarly work have focused on eating disorders, primary care aspects of psychiatry, family therapy, consultation–liaison psychiatry, stress, professional development and education in psychiatry and medicine, the development of practice guidelines, and, most recently, mental health services research. Dr. Yager has authored or coauthored more than 200 professional articles and book chapters, and has edited and coedited seven books, including *Teaching Psychiatry and Behavioral Science*, *The Future of Psychiatry as a Medical Specialty*, and *Special Problems in the Management of Eating Disorders*.

IOM STAFF

MICHAEL T. ABRAMS, M.P.H., is program officer with the Board on Neuroscience and Behavioral Health of the Institute of Medicine. He has served as study director for the present work and as program officer on a study of spinal cord injury research planning. He earned his masters of public health degree from The Johns Hopkins University (2000), where he focused his studies on childhood mental health disorders. From 1997 to 2001, he served as a junior faculty member in the Department of Psychiatry and Behavioral Sciences at The Johns Hopkins University School of Medicine. From 1994 to 2001, he was involved in and managed structural and functional neuroimaging experiments aimed at the elucidation of neuropathologies that underlie various genetic disorders affecting learning and language in children. From 1990 to 1994, he worked as a research assistant on a behavioral genetics investigation that focused on fragile X and Turner syndromes. He has authored or coauthored 25 peer-reviewed publications.

KATHLEEN M. PATCHAN is research assistant with the Board on Neuroscience and Behavioral Health. She has served in that capacity for the present study, and for a study on spinal cord injury research planning. She previously worked at the Center on Budget and Policy Priorities and the Congressional Research Service, focusing on Medicaid, the State Children's Health Insurance Program, and employer-sponsored health insurance. Ms. Patchan received bachelors degrees in cell and molecular biology and in history from the University of Maryland at College Park.

ANDREW M. POPE, Ph.D., is acting director of the Board on Neuroscience and Behavioral Health and director of the Board on Health Sciences Policy at the Institute of Medicine. With expertise in physiology and biochemistry, he focuses his work primarily on environmental and occupational influences on human health. Dr. Pope's previous research activities addressed the neuroendocrine and reproductive effects of various environmental substances on food-producing animals. During his tenure at the National Academy of Sciences and since 1989 at the Institute of Medicine, Dr. Pope has directed the preparation of numerous reports on topics that include injury control, disability prevention, biologic markers, neurotoxicology, indoor allergens, and the enhancement of environmental and occupational health content in medical and nursing school curricula. Most recently, Dr. Pope directed studies on National Institutes of Health priority-setting processes, fluid resuscitation practices in combat casualties, and organ procurement and transplantation.